IQBAL SINGH

CHAHAL

COVID WARRIOR

IQBAL SINGH CHAHAL

COVID WARRIOR

MINHAZ MERCHANT

AMARYLLIS

AMARYLLIS

An imprint of Manjul Publishing House Pvt. Ltd.
• C-16, Sector 3, Noida, Uttar Pradesh 201301, India
Website: www.manjulindia.com
Registered Office:
• 10, Nishat Colony, Bhopal 462 003 – India
Distribution Centres
Ahmedabad, Bengaluru, Bhopal, Kolkata, Chennai,
Hyderabad, Mumbai, Noida, Pune

Iqbal Singh Chahal: Covid Warrior by Minhaz Merchant

This edition first published in India in 2022
Third impression 2022

ISBN 978-93-5543-129-5

Printed and bound in India by Thomson Press (India) Ltd.

CONTENTS

FOREWORD

When the first case of Covid-19 hit Maharashtra, we knew that it was time for us to act. I was certain that this wasn't the last Covid-19 case in our country and at that moment I asked the urban local bodies to create field hospitals, known as Jumbo centres.

Along with medical facilities being ramped up, we started our movement towards a staggered lockdown until the prime minister announced the national lockdown on 24 March 2020.

Mumbai's global connect, population density and diversity demanded that the municipal corporation, the mayor and the people were supported by an administrative team leader who was dynamic and loved to lead the charge in the battlefield.

It was during the month of May 2020 that I appointed Iqbal Singh Chahal as the municipal commissioner of Mumbai. I told him that I was entrusting him with a great responsibility—Mumbai's Covid battle.

I am happy to note that Chahal and his team at the Municipal Corporation of Greater Mumbai (MCGM) have done an outstanding job under very difficult circumstances. Each day, our meetings and calls assured me that he was fully in control of the situation and ensured that we pushed our boundaries for the well-being of Mumbaikars who reposed their faith in us as an administration.

Be it decentralisation of ward war rooms, ambulance fleet management, Covid medicine management, or the natural disasters that we faced while battling Covid, Chahal has stood rock solid with me as an able team member who is willing to take responsibility and deliver what is promised.

It is due to this extremely passionate dedication of Chahal and the MCGM that what was initially dubbed as 'Mumbai's uphill task against Covid' is now simply and successfully called the 'Mumbai Model.'

I congratulate him on this effort to compile the experience of being a municipal commissioner of Mumbai, with all its marvels, delights of accomplishment and complexities of effort, and bringing forth Mumbai's rise against Covid-19.

This book gives a glimpse into the challenges converted to opportunities for Mumbai by Chahal, and the various emotions he felt of pain and joy, despair and hope that he at times voiced to me while managing Mumbai's Covid-19 challenge.

If I may say so, the story of the MCGM, led by Mayor Kishori Pednekar and Municipal Commissioner Chahal, truly signifies the 'spirit of Mumbai.'

Uddhav Balasaheb Thackeray
Chief Minister, Maharashtra
10 November 2021

AUTHOR'S NOTE

The Spanish Flu pandemic killed 50 million people worldwide between 1918 and 1920. A 100 years later, the Covid-19 pandemic has caused the deaths of over 5 million people globally, including more than half-a-million in India. The fatalities continue to rise, albeit in a gradually declining trajectory.

The origin of the SARS-CoV-2 coronavirus remains a mystery. The weight of evidence, however, points towards Wuhan, a high-tech city in China's Hubei province. Wuhan hosts several laboratories engaged in advanced biological research. Among the most prominent ones is the Wuhan Institute of Virology.

While the origin of Covid-19 is under renewed scrutiny by the World Health Organization (WHO) and scientists globally, the devastation it has caused in lives and livelihoods makes the pandemic the most lethal public health emergency in a century.

India, with its underfunded public health infrastructure and crowded urban spaces, was always likely to suffer disproportionately from a pandemic with the infectivity of Covid-19. And it did. Despite a total national lockdown that began on 25 March 2020 and lasted for over 2 months, India reeled under the impact of the Covid-19 pandemic. The economy ground to a halt. Hospitals could not cope with the influx of seriously ill patients. Dead bodies lay on pavements. The health infrastructure started crumbling and came close to a total collapse.

Mumbai was among the most severely affected cities in the pandemic. Over 50 per cent of Mumbai's population lives in slums. Physical distancing is impossible. And indeed, Mumbai took the brunt of the first wave of the pandemic as it rose up from Kerala and swept across the country.

Cometh the hour, cometh the man. As Mumbai became the country's Covid hotspot in March 2020 and struggled to control the rising tide of infections and a crippling shortage of hospital beds, Iqbal Singh Chahal was suddenly appointed municipal commissioner on 8 May 2020. Chief Minister Uddhav Thackeray told Chahal: 'This is your toughest assignment. If you succeed, it will be your success. If you fail, it will be my failure.' Mumbai was on fire; slums like Dharavi—the largest and most dense of slums in Asia—were reeling under the impact of the coronavirus.

An IAS officer of the 1989 batch, Chahal was no stranger to challenges. He took the new assignment head-on. On the morning of 9 May, less than 24 hours after he took charge as commissioner, Chahal inspected the Covid ICU of a major city hospital. Covid ICUs can be deathtraps even for those fully encased in sanitised Personal Protection Equipment (PPE) kits. Chahal didn't flinch. His mission began from a hospital Covid ICU and was followed by a 5-kilometre march the same day with his team through Dharavi's slum containment zones.

The mission would carry on through the first and second waves in 2020 and 2021 respectively as well as the Omicron triggered third wave. It would be speckled with risk-taking innovations by Chahal. He established 24 ward war rooms in place of one centralised control centre. There were over 27 other specific initiatives, including setting up several Jumbo field hospitals, demarcating containment zones in slum areas and requisitioning retired doctors from across the state to take care of the burgeoning patient caseload.

Chahal decided early on to run a transparent and open operation. Global media, ranging from the *Washington Post* to *The Economist*, lauded Mumbai's transparency. Chahal had set up a dashboard on a comprehensive website that provided data in real-time on the number of vacant hospital beds, Covid-positive cases and fatalities. By staying ahead of the narrative curve, fake news was swiftly countered. Chahal set up 30 groups on social media apps comprising 6,500 journalists, political leaders, IAS officers, diplomats, judges, activists and entertainment and sports celebrities to whom he messaged facts and data on Mumbai's battle against Covid-19.

I interviewed Chahal over 11 sessions, each lasting 3 hours. What emerges from this intense interaction spread over 8 months is a compelling account of how one of the world's most complex urban agglomerations dealt with the gravest public health crisis in a century.

Chahal's work as commissioner of the Municipal Corporation of Greater Mumbai (MCGM) has brought him international fame. He has received numerous awards and citations. In quite an extraordinary feat, Chahal received 11 international and national level awards over a period of just 12 months. A doctorate degree (*honoris causa*) was bestowed upon him by his alma mater, Thapar Institute of Engineering and Technology, Patiala, Punjab, a deemed university. His work has been widely appreciated and admired—from the Supreme Court of India to sitting US Congressmen. The innovations he employed to control the pandemic in Mumbai have been praised universally.

In this book, Chahal shares exclusively for the first time the full inside story of the personal and professional challenges he faced while combating Covid-19 and its variants, including Delta and Omicron. Post-vaccination, he believes, the city, the nation and the world must keep their guard up.

Researching and writing this book has been educative. For the reader, I hope it will prove to be an equally rewarding experience.

ACKNOWLEDGEMENTS

In a book tackling a subject of this complexity, it's important to acknowledge the professional cooperation I received at various levels. The first wave of Covid-19 had abated when I began researching and writing the manuscript. It wasn't long, however, before the far more infectious second wave engulfed India.

Globally, the resurgence of Covid-19 was devastating. Cities like New York and London reeled. In January 2021, Britain was laid low by a lethal surge in the pandemic. In a few short weeks between January and March 2021, British fatalities doubled to over 1.25 lakh. In the rest of Europe too, the pandemic's second wave struck hard, aborting travel and leading to a reimposition of strict lockdowns.

In the United States, though the vaccination roll out had progressed well, a fresh surge in cases in August and September 2021 took the count back to over 1 lakh a day though the mortality rate remained low. Vaccinations ensured that infections led to fewer deaths than in the pandemic's early phase.

In India, the second wave struck with ferocity. By April and May 2021, cases doubled, trebled and quadrupled. Deaths rose to over 4,000 a day—nearly four times the level of fatalities in the first wave. Oxygen shortages crippled health systems. Delhi was especially hard hit.

Mumbai escaped the worst of the devastation due to the lessons learnt in the first wave and the innovations the MCGM, led by Commissioner Iqbal Singh Chahal, had instituted. Many systems were now on autopilot. Mumbai registered one of the lowest mortality rates (0.8 per cent) for a comparable global city anywhere.

It was during the challenging second wave that this book took final shape. I would like to place on record my gratitude to Commissioner Chahal for sparing dozens of hours over several months going over every aspect of how Mumbai confronted the Covid-19 pandemic.

The wealth of research material I was given access to makes this book a historically important record of how the city fought the biggest public health crisis in a century.

I am grateful to various people, some of whom wish to remain unnamed, who helped in numerous ways to make this book possible and bring a complex project to fruition.

I remain deeply grateful too to my family, especially, my wife Kahini, for her patience and support during this period. Last but not the least, I would like to thank my assistant, Rukshana Kumar, whose diligence right through the project was exemplary.

I hope readers derive as much satisfaction from reading this book as I did researching and writing it.

ONE

CHASING THE VIRUS

Covid-19 struck India by stealth. The first positive case was discovered in Kerala on 30 January 2020. A period of quietude followed.

Iqbal Singh Chahal, a senior IAS officer, was at the time posted in Mantralaya, the Maharashtra government's official seat of power. Sitting today in his high-ceilinged, British-built municipal commissioner's office at the headquarters of the Municipal Corporation of Greater Mumbai (MCGM) located in an imposing heritage building opposite the Chhatrapati Shivaji Maharaj Terminus (CSMT), Chahal recalls: 'It was around 11 March 2020 when the Indian government recognised the enormous danger the coronavirus posed.'

The first case appeared in Mumbai on 16 March 2020. 'It's important to remember,' Chahal points out, 'that the first lockdown was announced by the Maharashtra government on 21 March 2020, much before the national lockdown. Fortunately, I was posted at that time in Mantralaya as principal secretary in the Maharashtra government's Urban Development Department. The very next day, after Maharashtra announced the lockdown, a janata curfew was proclaimed by Prime Minister Narendra Modi on 22 March. Immediately after the janata curfew—which of course was voluntary—a national lockdown was imposed from 25 March. It continued, with periodic extensions, till

31 May. As soon as the 25 March lockdown set in, the Maharashtra government decided to appoint me as nodal officer for monitoring the Covid situation in the state as principal secretary. My office was situated in close proximity to then Chief Secretary Ajoy Mehta's office in Mantralaya.'

When the first wave of the Covid-19 pandemic broke out in Maharashtra, few realised its gravity. Chahal reflects today: 'A series of discussions were being held on the likely magnitude of this pandemic. No one had imagined its intensity and longevity. Our generation, or the generation of our fathers and grandfathers, had never seen such a global pandemic. The last pandemic, the Spanish Flu, struck in 1918. So it was very difficult to imagine the havoc a global pandemic could wreak. Terms like quarantine, or even pandemic, had rarely been used in decades.'

The first hint of unprecedented measures to combat the pandemic came on 24 March 2020. 'That afternoon I attended a meeting at Chief Minister Uddhav Thackeray's official residence, Varsha, on Malabar Hill,' recalls Chahal. 'As we entered the meeting hall, I spotted Praveen Pardeshi, then the city's municipal commissioner. None of us knew the magnitude of the problem. Everyone thought that we would have one or two lockdowns and the matter would be over in a month or so. At 8.00 pm on 24 March, hours after our meeting had ended at the CM's residence, Prime Minister Narendra Modi went on national television. He called for a 3-week total national lockdown starting midnight that day. The lockdown was extended for another 3 weeks. In all, the country was locked down from 24 March till May 2020. Citizens had received less than 4 hours notice to prepare for what would prove to be a traumatic period for all Indians.'

At 8.00 pm sharp, on 24 March, the prime minister emerged grim-faced from an unscheduled cabinet meeting. He began his address to the nation: 'Namaskaar! My dear fellow citizens, today, once again, I am in your midst to discuss the corona global pandemic.

'All of you are listening to and watching news items regarding the pandemic situation around the world. All of you are also witnessing how the most advanced countries of the world have been rendered absolutely helpless by this pandemic. It is not that these countries are not putting in adequate efforts or that they lack resources. The coronavirus is spreading at such a rapid pace that despite all the preparations and efforts, these countries are finding it hard to manage the crisis. The opinion of experts has proved that there is only one way to effectively deal with the coronavirus—social distancing. That is, maintain physical distance from others and stay within the confines of your home. There is no other method or way to escape the coronavirus. If we want to restrict the spread of the coronavirus, we will have to break its chain of infection. Carelessness of a few, ill-conceived notions of a few, can put you, your children, your parents, your family, your friends, the entire country in grave jeopardy. It will be impossible to estimate the price India will have to pay if this carelessness continues.

'Friends, in the last 2 days, several parts of the country have been put under lockdown. These efforts by the state governments should be taken with utmost sincerity. In light of inputs from health sector experts and the experience of other countries, the nation is taking a very important decision today. From midnight tonight onwards, the entire country, please listen carefully, the entire country shall go under complete lockdown. In order to protect the country, and each of its citizens, from midnight tonight, a full ban is being imposed on people from stepping out of their homes. All the states in the country, all the union territories, each district, each municipality, each village, each locality, is being put under lockdown.

'This is a necessary step in the decisive fight against the coronavirus pandemic. The nation will have to certainly pay an economic cost because of this lockdown. However, to save the life of each and every Indian is mine, the government of India's, each state government's, each local unit's, topmost priority. Hence, it is my plea to you to continue staying wherever you are right now in the country. Considering the circumstances at present, this lockdown will last 21 days. The next 21 days are of critical importance for us. As per health experts, a period of at least 21 days is extremely critical to break the infection chain of the coronavirus.

'If the situation is not handled in these 21 days, the country and your family could go back 21 years. If the situation is not handled in these 21 days, several families will get devastated forever. Hence, you must forget what going out means for the next 21 days. Stay inside your home, stay inside your home, and do just one thing—stay inside your home. 21 days of lockdown is a long time, but it is equally essential for your safety and that of your family. I am confident that every Indian will not only successfully fight this difficult situation but also emerge victorious. Take care of yourself and your loved ones. Jai Hind!'

In the event, the 21-day national lockdown was the precursor of the trauma that Covid-19, as the SARS-CoV-2 coronavirus was later named by the World Health Organization (WHO), would inflict on the world.

Chahal was given the responsibility to monitor 27 municipal corporations and 34 collectorates across Maharashtra by then chief secretary, Ajoy Mehta. 'My job,' he says reflectively, 'was complex. I created a file on Google Drive with 61 officers—34 collectors and 27 municipal chiefs. Early every morning, I received data from these 61 officers across the state on the situation monitored the previous day.'

The information flow was precise: how many people had tested positive, district-wise and municipal corporation-wise. 'Then there was contact tracing,' says Chahal. 'If someone was positive in Malegaon or Sangli or Pune, I had to coordinate with the collectors and municipal commissioners to trace their contacts—high-risk and low-risk too. We collated and entered the complete data in the file on Google Drive daily and presented it to the state government.'

Hospitals were divided into specific categories. The Maharashtra government assigned the task to Chahal. 'We placed our hospitals across Maharashtra, covering 12.5 crore (125 milllion) people, into four categories,' recounts Chahal. 'That categorisation was done personally by me for the 61 municipal corporations and collectorates in the state.'

The process was completed between 25 March and 15 April 2020 during the first 3-week phase of the total nationwide lockdown. Chahal believes that the strict lockdown gave the city and the MCGM critical time to prepare. 'If the complete lockdown had not been in place,' Chahal affirms, 'there would have been complete chaos.' He adds sombrely: 'Lockdowns may or may not have controlled the spread of Covid-19 in the first wave when we knew little about the coronavirus. But they gave us time to prepare. We told the collectors to categorise their hospitals into four parts: Covid Care Centres (CCC), Dedicated Covid Health Centres (DCHC), Dedicated Covid Hospitals (DCH) and non-Covid Hospitals at the district and taluka level, both government and private. First, we had to create Covid Care Centres in them. These Covid Care Centres, which we called triple C, would be managed only by ayurvedic doctors or homeopathic doctors. There would be no MBBS doctors there.

'These Covid Care Centres were created to take care of asymptomatic positive cases. Suppose somebody is found to be Covid-positive but he lives in a slum. He does not have an independent bathroom or an independent bedroom. He could spread the virus to his family members. He should therefore be escorted out and put in a CCC. Since he does not have symptoms, he does not need oxygen, medication or a ventilator. He just needs to be kept under observation. So we told the 27 municipal commissioners across Maharashtra at our meetings that they had to create sufficient numbers of Covid Care Centres where these large numbers of asymptomatic cases would be placed. They would be monitored there for 10 days. Each Covid Care Centre would have an ambulance linked to a major hospital and it would be parked right outside the CCC.'

Since knowledge about the virus was still limited, Chahal had to nuance his strategy in the early days of the pandemic. Innovative measures needed to be taken. 'The easiest way to create Covid Care Centres was to take over dharamshalas, mangal karyalas, small one or two star hotels, and so on,' he says. 'In Mumbai, we created 48,000 beds by requisitioning 187 hotels. If anyone was found Covid-positive, he was sent to a Covid Care Centre and monitored there. Suppose after the third or fifth day, he started showing symptoms like fever and breathlessness, then the ambulance driver, dressed in a PPE kit, would take him to a DCHC. In case he did not develop any symptoms, he was tested on the seventh day and again on the tenth day. If found negative, he was discharged and sent home. If the results did not come negative on the tenth day, we did a third test on the fourteenth day.'

The second category of care centres that Chahal put in place in the fraught early days of the pandemic comprised Dedicated Covid Health Centres. The DCHCs had one MBBS doctor, an oxygen facility and a paramedical staff. They did not have an Intensive Care Unit (ICU), operation theatre or specialist doctors. The DCHCs were akin to municipal dispensaries or district hospitals which did not have operation theatres and ICUs. They, however, had an oxygen facility near each bed. If a patient tested positive for Covid, was feeling breathless and had fever, he was driven directly into a DCHC. Doctors administered oxygen and minimum medication to take care of the symptoms. If the patient's symptoms worsened, the ambulance stationed at the DCHC took him to a Dedicated Covid Hospital (for example, the private Breach Candy Hospital, or the public Nair Hospital).

The state's municipal commissioners and administrators now created a third category of care centres—Dedicated Covid Hospitals.

Chahal explains the strategy: 'These Dedicated Covid Hospitals had ICUs, ventilators, operation theatres, oxygen beds and dialysis beds. We also instituted a fourth category of non-Covid centres like Breach Candy Hospital which would have both a Covid centre and a non-Covid centre. For example, if a non-Covid person met with an accident and had a skull fracture or suffered a heart attack, such patients also needed to be attended to. The non-Covid hospitals were meant for them. Thus the entire state of Maharashtra—all 245 municipalities, 35 districts and 27 municipal corporations—were included in this classification. It was the Union government which suggested this classification.'

These were still the initial weeks of the pandemic. But quick action gave Maharashtra—and in particular Mumbai—an early edge in tackling the virus during the first wave. 'We prepared a data bank online: names of hospitals, the nodal person there, his telephone number and name,' says Chahal. 'We flashed all this information through TV channels, digital platforms, social media and word of mouth so that every citizen was aware of these facilities in the event of contracting a coronavirus infection. All this took place between 1 April and 30 April 2020 during the total national lockdown. There was not a single day I was sitting at home. I came to my Mantralaya office every day, often working late into the night. Mantralaya was at that time working with a skeleton staff and services.'

Chahal was given charge of all the state's hospitals as well as overall Covid reporting. Another IAS officer at secretary level was put in charge of foodgrains supply. Other secretaries monitored the distribution of food packets in slum areas, logistics, migrant labourers and inter-state train movements. Yet another secretary coordinated with state-level secretaries to ensure that everything functioned smoothly during the national lockdown.

Having assumed responsibility at an early stage of the pandemic for the frontal tasks of monitoring hospitals, Covid centre classification and Covid reporting, Chahal got a bird's eye view of the coronavirus spreading rapidly across the city and the state. He recalls: 'I absorbed first-hand knowledge of contact tracing and high- and low-risk contacts. Two critical events took place now. They would have important consequences on the spread of the coronavirus in Maharashtra and beyond.

'First, between 1 January and 22 March 2020, 2.70 lakh international passengers landed at the Mumbai airport. It became the root cause of Mumbai's first Covid-19 wave. Between 1 February and 22 March 2020 alone, 1.75 lakh people disembarked at the Mumbai airport. The 22 March flight was the last one from abroad. After that the lockdown set in and all international travel was stopped. But some of the passengers who had arrived were already Covid-positive. They had come from Europe, especially from Italy, and the Middle East. They spread the coronavirus like wildfire in Mumbai. Many of these passengers travelled to other cities in Maharashtra and across the rest of India. If we had stopped international flights by 1 February 2020, then the first wave of the pandemic would not have struck India in the way it did. The coronavirus came from abroad. India did not have this virus. Covid-19 started in China, went to Europe, the Middle East and then came to India.'

The government gave Chahal the additional task of tracing passengers who had arrived at Mumbai and could be Covid-19 carriers. 'It was a Herculean task,' admits Chahal. 'My main challenge was to get a list from the immigration authorities of the 2.70 lakh passengers who had arrived in Mumbai on international flights between 1 January and 22 March 2020 and track them down through telephone numbers. We managed to track down nearly 50,000 people. There are 24 wards in Mumbai. We created a Google doc for 24 ward officers. When the immigration list of those 2.70 lakh passengers came to us, we saw that

49,000 people had Mumbai addresses. The rest were spread across Maharashtra. The addresses of these 49,000 people who were from Mumbai were given to different wards in Mumbai. Each ward had around 2,000 names. These 2,000 names were split and analysed by ward officers. We told each ward to create 10 squads. They had to go house-to-house identifying these people. That's how we tracked all the passengers. Around 200 people from the passenger list had become Covid-positive by this time. They were shifted to hospitals for treatment. Sadly, some of them passed away during this very difficult period.'

On 2 April 2020 the Maharashtra government received a report from the Union home ministry in Delhi that 2,400 Tablighis would shortly enter the state. Chahal was again given the responsibility of tracking these 2,400 potential Covid carriers. 'We did manage to track a lot of them,' says Chahal. 'In fact, Maharashtra has several districts like Latur, Beed, Aurangabad and Osmanabad with a relatively large Muslim population. When these Tablighis arrived in Maharashtra, the number of Covid cases started rising in those areas. The entry of the coronavirus in Vidharba and Marathawada during the first wave was partly due to the Tablighis.'

As the public health crisis intensified, the Narendra Modi government regularly dispatched a team of Covid specialists to Maharashtra and other parts of India. 'When the Centre's Covid team came to Mumbai in the first week of May 2020,' Chahal says, 'Chief Minister Uddhav Thackeray ordered a video conference with the state's municipal commissioners and collectors. I was present in the conference as principal secretary, urban development. I placed all the facts before the authorities, including information about symptomatic and asymptomatic patients in various districts. I listened carefully to feedback from the Centre's Covid team after it had visited various parts of Maharashtra.'

The Delhi team gave a scathing report against the MCGM. It said it had inspected various containment zones within the sprawling Dharavi slum. Team members had asked the residents in the slum's containment zones if MCGM workers visited their homes on a regular basis and checked their temperature and oxygen levels. The answers were blunt: MCGM health workers came to the exit gates of the containment zone and merely filled out forms as they were fearful of entering the slum's containment areas. They then reported back claiming that they had completed their job. But in effect, surveillance of the spread of Covid-19 in Dharavi was not taking place. The team also complained that mortality data was not being updated at crematoriums by the local Covid-19 monitoring teams.

The Centre's visiting health task force provided its findings to Chief Minister Thackeray before returning to Delhi. The Modi government was visibly unhappy with the situation in Maharashtra. In April 2020, Mumbai had just 3,700 Covid beds for a population of 15 million that fell under the MCGM's jurisdiction. The virus was spreading exponentially. People were dying before being admitted to a hospital. The city's health infrastructure was clearly too weak to deal with a pandemic of this magnitude. As many as 21 public interest litigations (PILs) were filed before the Bombay High Court by May 2020 demanding dismissal of the Maha Vikas Aghadi (MVA) state government. Deaths in Mumbai climbed to almost 100 a day in May 2020.

Before leaving for Delhi, the centre's team team members also noted that crematorium registers in Mumbai were not available. Nobody quite knew how many people had died of Covid. Chahal describes the grim scenario: 'They thought that the state government was trying to hide facts and not updating the data. They also observed that food packets were not reaching labourers during the national lockdown. Initially, testing capacity was limited. So a Covid test would be done only against a prescription as there were only two labs then for testing. The centre's team noted that when slum dwellers came to a flu clinic with a temperature and a cough, they would be prescribed paracetamol instead of a Covid test and appropriate medical care. The patients would consume paracetamol and their condition would worsen. Often, they would die. The Union government team told Chief Minister Thackeray that this was a dangerous situation. You cannot suppress Covid symptoms through paracetamol, they warned. This became an issue as the team from Delhi claimed that the Maharashtra government was trying to suppress Covid figures by giving patients paracetamol.

The Thackeray government moved swiftly to remedy matters. Alok Deshpande reported in *The Hindu*[1]:

> 'The Maharashtra government's health department has set up two committees to analyse the deaths of patients and measures to reduce fatalities. While one committee will concentrate on Mumbai, the other will focus on the rest of Maharashtra. According to Health Minister Rajesh Tope, in the case of death of a Covid-19 patient, the chief of the hospital will provide information on the patient's treatment, medical history and other details to the committee via video conferencing. Principal Secretary (Health) Pradeep Vyas has communicated this to all district collectors, municipal commissioners and district medical chiefs. A seven-member committee will look specifically at cases in and around Mumbai since the number is high here. "The committee will analyse the reasons behind the deaths due to the coronavirus and based on that measures could be suggested to reduce the number of deaths," said Mr Tope.

'Thackeray also announced a task force of specialist doctors to be

[1] 15 April 2020.

chaired by Dr Sanjay Oak. It included a number of specialist doctors[2] from the private sector, including Dr Zahir Udwadia (Hinduja Hospital), Dr Santoshi Nagvekar (Lilavati Hospital), Dr Kedar Toraskar (Wockhardt Hospital), Dr Rahul Pandit (Fortis Hospital), Dr Nitin Karnik (Lokmanya Tilak Hospital, Sion), Dr Zahir Virani (Prince Aly Khan Hospital) and Dr Om Srivastav (Kasturba, Jaslok). Dr Praveen Bangar (KEM Hospital) was the convener. Deshpande reported that the task force will establish a patient management protocol for serious and critically ill patients. It will recommend specialist doctors and healthcare support staff in critical care hospitals, a suitable drug protocol to maintain uniformity in treating critically-ill patients, and the criteria and logistics requirement to transfer critical patients.

The Thackeray government was now becoming increasingly concerned about the impact of Covid-19 on Mumbai's slums. Dharavi was in the eye of the Covid-19 storm. It would play an important role in the recognition Mumbai received in the global media for its successful battle to contain Covid-19 in one of the world's most complex urban agglomerations.

Unexpectedly, in the middle of the first wave of the pandemic, the MCGM got a new municipal commissioner. Chahal leans back on a sofa in his spacious office as he recalls the rapid-fire events that unfolded on 8 May 2020: 'I was attending office every day in Mantralaya. On the morning of 8 May at around 10 am, Chief Minister Uddhav Thackeray phoned me at home just as I was about to leave for office. He said that the government was planning to appoint two commissioners for the MCGM—one Covid commissioner and one normal municipal commissioner. Praveen Pardeshi would continue as the municipal commissioner and I would be the Covid commissioner.

[2]Pooja Biraia Jaiswal, *The Week*, 14 April 2020.

'I told the chief minister that I was honoured by his offer. I have been in government service for over 30 years. I know that unless you have complete control over your team, it doesn't work. Accountability cannot come without power. Two commissioners would create a lot of confusion. I told the CM that this system will not work as the staff will have divided loyalty. I said to the CM, with utmost respect, that if he wanted me to do Covid monitoring, then instead of monitoring the entire state of Maharashtra as I was then tasked with doing, I could do a close monitoring of just Mumbai city. I thought this arrangement would work. I would travel ward to ward, hospital to hospital, start collecting data and every morning I would report to the chief minister. But I said to the CM that if you want me to control the situation, then I should act as the leader and declare war on Covid. There has to be only one person in charge.'

The morning phone call between Thackeray and Chahal lasted for just under 25 minutes. 'If he put me in charge, I assured the CM, I would try my best,' recalls Chahal. 'The CM said he would think about it but did not say yes. After that the CM interacted with then Chief Secretary Ajoy Mehta. Later on, at about 2.30 pm, the CM called me again. He said he had discussed the matter with the chief secretary. 'Chahal, we are issuing orders to appoint you as municipal commissioner,' he told me in his usual brisk, businesslike manner. He asked me where I was. I told him I was just a few minutes away from Mantralaya. The CM told me to proceed immediately to Mantralaya and meet the chief secretary. I could choose my entire team.

'It was 2.30 pm, 8 May. I still remember the date and time. The MCGM traditionally has four additional commissioners. They are all senior IAS officers. The CM asked me to select the four I wanted as the Covid situation in the city was getting out of control. I met Chief Secretary Ajoy Mehta at around 3.00 pm. I informed him about my talk with the CM. Mehta advised me to pick my four additional commissioners carefully. I rang up the CM at 5.00 pm and briefed him about the officers I had selected. I asked for Ashwini Bhide and Sanjeev Jaiswal, both very competent IAS officers. He gave me the go ahead. The orders were issued around 6.30 pm. At 7.00 pm sharp, I entered this chamber.'

Chahal looks up at the high ornate ceiling in the office of the municipal commissioner that harks back to the colonial era. His voice rises a pitch: 'I had told the staff that I would be arriving shortly at this office and we would hold a meeting. All ward officers needed to be present along with the medical officer of health (MoH), senior doctors, deputy commissioners, joint commissioners and additional commissioners. There are about 120 of us. All this took place on the evening of 8 May. I had called the ward meeting within half an hour of my appointment. The physical meeting at our headquarters lasted almost 3 hours. It finished around midnight. In those initial Covid-19 days, no one held physical meetings. The national lockdown was still on. Everyone held virtual meetings. My father, Lt. Colonel Man Singh Chahal (Retd.), an army officer, always told me that for important meetings one must have eyeball-to-eyeball contact. Unless that face-to-face contact takes place, the meeting will not deliver results.

'At 7.30 pm, when I arrived at the MCGM office, there were about 120-plus officers in the hall adjoining this chamber. I knew the subject of this meeting well. I knew what was tracing, tracking, quarantine, treatment, high-risk contact, low-risk contact as I had been involved in the Covid battle over the past 2 months. Otherwise, I would have wasted many days learning about what was happening. In this meeting I made a couple of points that I will never forget in my life.

'First, I addressed the entire team and told them that on this day, 8 May 2020, Mumbai has 11,000 cummulative positive cases and New York has 50,000 daily positive cases. I encouraged my team and told them that I knew they were being criticised by the media, by the courts, by the Opposition, by the central government. But this should not be seen as a setback for us. We have 11,000 positive case. Look at other cities. New York was recording 50,000 positive cases every day despite having half the population of Mumbai. I told my team they had done a great job for the past more than 45 days, starting from 20 March 2020. But now what we face is the beginning of the problem. Covid-19 is not going to go away for years. This job is not going to be completed in one month or two or three.'

Even Chahal would not have known as the first wave of the coronavirus washed over Mumbai, just how long the battle would last as wave after wave struck the country with deadly mutant variants of the virus.

Meanwhile, Chahal instructed the officers and workers in his team who had comorbidities to submit their names that very night. He did not want to risk their lives. 'I told them that I am a marathon runner, an experienced swimmer, a yoga instructor, I have high body immunity and in the last 10 years I have not had even a bad throat,' says Chahal. 'I had confidence in myself that I would tide over the crisis. My immunity would help me. Immunity is the best weapon against Covid. But I said to my team members that if anyone had undergone a bypass surgery or had kidney problems or was on dialysis or was a diabetic, then they should submit their names tonight or the first thing tomorrow morning as I did not want to risk their health. I would put them on other assignments which did not involve frontline work. Our mantra was "to perform or perish" and it applied to the entire team, including me, the commissioner.'

Chahal said there was no complusion if any team member did not want to fight this war. They would be eased out from the frontline. At the time, in the second week of May 2020, as the coronavirus raged amidst a strict national lockdown, a majority of the MCGM's 1,08,000 employees were sequestered at home with full pay. Chahal becomes thoughtful as he casts his mind back to those early days of the pandemic: 'I told my staff that none of us will sit in these AC rooms. We have been criticised for not entering the slums and containment zones. So now, starting from the commissioner, no one will be sitting in their chambers. Morning to evening we will be in the field. I had realised by then that this was going to prove to be one of the most difficult assignments of my career.'

In the early hours of 9 May, around 1.30 am, shortly after he had reached home following the grueling 3-hour meeting at the MCGM headquarters with 120 members of his team, Chahal received a phone call. It was Chief Minister Uddhav Thackeray. He told the newly appointed municipal commissioner that he had taken on a tough assignment. Chahal briefed him on the day's work: 'I told the CM that I had taken charge last evening and had conducted a meeting with my team. Today, I was planning to go to Nair Hospital and then to Dharavi. He told me to be careful as the coronavirus was spreading fast. Several health workers had lost their lives. But he also said something which I will never forget. He told me that he had given me a very critical and important responsibility. One cannot imagine what kind of powers you have with this kind of responsibility, he said. This chair is so powerful that your conduct has to be of the highest order.

'The CM told me that if you succeed in this near impossible task, then that success will be all yours. But if you fail, then it will be the CM's failure. That statement hit my heart and soul like a bullet. I was carried away by the trust the CM had placed in me. I assured him, come what may, I will do my best. I don't care even if I lose my life. At that point in time, Covid was spreading so rapidly that if the situation would have worsened and more people would have died, then the CM would have had to resign.'

Chahal received more than 1,000 messages on his mobile phone on taking over as the new municipal commissioner. Many of them exclaimed that he had been put in the most difficult chair in India at that time. His father-in-law, Ajit Singh Chatha, the former chief secretary of Punjab, called him and asked whether he should congratulate him or not? Chahal was selected for one of the senior most assignments in the state IAS cadre even though his name stood at no. 33 in senority of serving IAS officers in the state. He says he now had only one option: to succeed at any cost.

Chahal is visibly emotional as he recalls that late night conversation with Uddhav Thackeray. A few days later, Chief Secretary Ajoy Mehta told Chahal that one of the "most senior" politicians of the state, on hearing of Chahal's likely appointment as municipal commissioner, had confided in Mehta: 'Generals are not changed during a war.' Mehta had replied: 'We have already lost the war the way Covid-19 has spread in Mumbai. That is the reason we have to change the general.'

Chahal got down to work early on the morning of 9 May. He phoned Dr Gautam Bhansali, a senior consultant physician at Bombay Hospital. 'I called him at around 7.30 am,' Chahal recalls. 'I asked him to come home as I wanted to go to Nair Hospital's Covid ICU ward. He would have to help me wear the PPE kit, to dress and undress, as I did not know how to do these things. The first precaution I took was to take Dr Bhansali along. We started at 9.00 am. We changed into PPE kits. We then went directly into the Covid ICU ward at Nair Hospital. Those days things were so bad, with hundreds of deaths daily, that nobody other than fully protected doctors and nurses would dare enter a Covid ICU. At Nair Hospital, there were 45 patients in the Covid ICU; 10 patients were on ventilators and 35 patients were on oxygen, struggling for life. Around 10 doctors and nurses and a couple of ward boys were present.

'I entered the Covid ICU ward with the additional municipal commissioner, the dean of the hospital and Dr Gautam Bhansali. We did not want crowding there. I went to the bedside of all 45 patients and spoke to the doctors about their health as some of the patients could not speak due to oxygen masks or ventilators. I spoke to the nurses and gave them my mobile number in case of an emergency. I interacted with the ward boys, appreciating their work. I checked on the availability of medicines and other issues concerning the ICU.'

Chahal and Dr Bhansali spent 53 minutes in Nair Hospital's Covid ICU ward. They later gave a presentation in the dean's office for half an hour about their observations of the Covid situation in the hospital. 'After finishing our visit at Nair Hospital,' Chahal recounts, 'we carefully removed our PPE kits and went straight to Dharavi at around 11.30 am. I asked the ward officer in charge there about which was the most infected pocket in Dharavi. Mukund Nagar, he said, was the most infected. There were 250 cases in that containment zone. Again we put on our full PPE kits. We walked along the slum for 5 kilometres. I have been running half-marathons since 2004—a total of 17 so far in all. But walking even 5 kilometres in Dharavi's most infected pocket was a different matter altogether.

'In Mukund Nagar, we entered public toilets, shanty houses, talked to shopkeepers and visited medical shops. I asked people about the delivery of food packets and whether their toilets were being sanitised. In Dharavi, 200 people share one toilet, so one can imagine how dangerously and rapidly Covid-19 could spread. We decided during that visit to Dharavi on 9 May that it was crucial to address the toilet issue. This is the point where maximum infections occur. Going to Mukund Nagar was a great learning experience. I saw first-hand the issues people were facing in the early months of the pandemic and whether health workers were stepping up to help, whether adequate testing was taking place, and if tracing was being done. In May 2020, there were 8-10 deaths in Dharavi alone every single day.'

From Dharavi, Chahal went straight home. 'In my flat, there is a fire refuge area, so I went there first and discarded everything, my PPE suit and my clothes,' Chahal recalls. 'I threw away my infected clothes since they posed a serious danger to my family after my nearly hour-long visit to the Covid ICU ward in Nair Hospital and the walk through Dharavi's infected bylanes. So I wore a towel and dashed straight to the bathroom for a shower. I did not touch a single item in the house as the fear of Covid-19 at the time was at its peak.'

That fear would multiply a year later as an even more infectious wave of the coronavirus swept through India, targeting Mumbai the rest of Maharashtra first. But way back in May 2020, the virus had already emerged as the most serious public health emergency in decades.

On 9 May Chahal's first full day as municipal commissioner, a man died of Covid while still in an autorickshaw in Dadar, central Mumbai. 3 dead bodies were found on a nearby pavement and one on the road divider. 5 other dead bodies lay unattended in public areas. Covid-19 was taking a heavy toll on the city, especially on the poor and the unprotected. Chahal went to other Covid hotspots over the next few days. He visited slums across Mumbai. The continuing learning experience for him and his team proved to be a game changer in the city's strategy to tackle both the first and the more virulent second wave of the Covid-19 pandemic.

Frenetic activity now followed. 'From 10 May,' Chahal says, 'I began to take multiple Zoom meetings every day. Through the whole day there were multiple things happening. It was tough to keep track of time. One day, when I was attending a cabinet meeting, I didn't remember what date it was that day. I had to ask my colleague about the day and date. That was the situation at the time. We were working round the clock. I was sleeping in the office. I did not go home on most days. On 10 May, I told my wife and son to move to Chandigarh. The situation was very bad in Mumbai and I did not want to infect them as I was constantly meeting with Covid-positive patients. They would remain in Chandigarh for the next several months.

'After they left, I went all out in the battle against the coronavirus. I was alone at home. I could sleep in my office for 2 or 3 days at a stretch. At home there was now no risk of infecting others. I used to have regular meetings by video conference with my core team which included 24 ward officers, 7 deputy commissioners and four additional commissioners. On 10 May, I told my team that we were going to coin a new policy: *chase the virus*. The virus was chasing people and many had already died. The number of infected people had also shot up. By the end of May 2020, it had risen to 40,000. Deaths were nearly 100 per day. So now it was our turn to chase the virus.'

Through the summer of 2020, the tidings were grim. A report[3] by Abhirup Roy, Devjyot Ghosal and Aaditya Kalra captured the unfolding human tragedy in Mumbai in graphic detail:

> 'When Manit Parikh's mother tested positive for the coronavirus, she was rushed by ambulance to Mumbai's private Lilavati Hospital, but officials told the family no critical-care beds were available. 5 hours and dozens of phone calls later, the family found a bed for her at the private Bombay Hospital. A day later, on 18 May Parikh's 92-year-old diabetic grandfather had breathing difficulties at home and was taken to the city's Breach Candy Hospital, another top private facility, but there were no beds. "My dad was pleading with them," Parikh told Reuters. "They said they didn't have a bed, not even a normal bed." Later that day, they found a bed at Bombay Hospital but his grandfather died hours later. His test results showed he was infected with the virus.

'Parikh said he believes the delays contributed to his grandfather's death. Officials at Lilavati and Bombay Hospital declined to speak with Reuters. Representatives of Breach Candy Hospital did not respond to requests for comment. For years, India's booming private hospitals

[3]Reuters, 18 May 2020.

have taken some of the strain off the country's underfunded and dilapidated public health network, but the ordeal of Parikh's family suggests that as the coronavirus cases explode in India, even private facilities are at risk of being overrun.'

Chahal's team, meanwhile, took the virus head-on. They entered the slums, went to the homes of slum dwellers and tested them. Anyone found positive was taken to a Covid Care Centre and 15 of his or her close relatives, friends and neighbours placed in quarantine. 'At this stage, we decided to requisition hotels and scale up quarantine beds,' says Chahal. 'It took us 7 days but we requisitioned 187 hotels, including two-, three-, four- and five-star hotels. We paid them accordingly: ₹1,000 per day for two-star hotels, ₹1,500 for three-star hotels, ₹2,000 for four-star hotels and ₹2,500 for five-star hotels. The hotels included food in this cost. They were empty anyway so they welcomed our proposal. By 20 May, we had created 48,000 beds in quarantine hotels and 24,000 beds in public places we had dubbed triple C—Covid Care Centres. Triple Cs included dharamshalas, mangal karalayas, halls, clinics and dispensaries. Those who were in touch with Covid-positive patients but were asymptomatic themselves were put up in hotels or triple Cs.'

There was initial resistance to forced quarantining from relatives and neighbours of Covid-positive patients. 'But later,' says Chahal, 'when they saw that they were well-looked-after with free boarding and lodging for 10 days in three-star and four-star hotels and we were sanitising their homes, the reluctance subsided. We started moving 30,000 people a week to cut them off from the virus. They were moved to cleaner, sanitised areas. If these 30,000 people had been left behind in the same households as their Covid-positive relatives at the peak of the first wave, they could have created 3,00,000 Covid-positive cases later on.

'This system was not put in place anywhere else in the world. First, you must have a large pool of quarantine beds and sufficient personnel and infrastructure to pick people up and house them. We were the only city to follow an active chase the virus policy. Around 1.44 lakh people were moved out in the first few weeks of the pandemic. For 10 days we monitored them for Covid-19. Tests were conducted. If they were negative, we sent them home; if they were positive, we sent them to a hospital. Around 10 per cent tested positive and they were moved to hospitals with oxygen beds. The remaining people returned to their sanitised environment.

'This was one part of our intense chase the virus strategy. The second part was sanitising public toilets not once a day but six times a day. Every toilet—nearly 1,000 in all—in the city's slums started getting sanitised six times daily. And that protocol continues even today. We hired professional agencies to do the sanitisation. To ensure seamless monitoring, I announced that I wanted 100 per cent physical attendance. The MCGM was the first institution in Mumbai to have 100 per cent staff attendance from May-June 2020. We spoke to the CM several times a day, reporting to him on the progress made in real-time.'

Meanwhile, top corporates stepped in to help with food and protective equipment. Since hotels were shut, doctors and nurses lived at various Taj Group hotels. The Tata Group donated high-quality food packets to health workers. Taj Hotel supplied thousands of meals every day. Chahal commends the Tatas: 'Tatas helped us with 58,000 room nights, 3 million meals, the creation of 600 additional beds in municipal hospitals, 20 ambulances, 73,000 PPE kits, 1.7 lakh masks and RT-PCR test kits. Taj Air Stats were providing meals to doctors and paramedical staff in major municipal hospitals. All this came free of cost from the Tatas. Ratan Tata is a legend, a class apart. He would call me after every few days and ask me if we needed anything else. I salute him. Besides the Tatas, other major corporate houses like Reliance Industries, Brittania, the Aditya Birla Group and the Anand Mahindra Group among others also greatly helped the MCGM.'

The MCGM's early steps helped it prepare for the second wave in February 2021. The sanitisation protocol had collateral benefits as well. In 2020-21, the city had zero malaria and dengue deaths. There are normally a 100 deaths in Mumbai every year from these serious illnesses. The success in containing the pandemic in Dharavi, meanwhile, became a *cause célèbre*.

Newspaper reporter Sanjana Bhalerao noted[4]: 'Dharavi, the 2.5-square kilometre slum sprawl, which had emerged as a Covid-19 hotspot in Mumbai by mid-April, and had the MCGM deeply worried, has witnessed a steady decline in the number of new cases in June. On Saturday, addition to cases was in single digits for the first time since the area reported its first case on 1 April.

'On 1 April, Dharavi reported its first Covid-19 case and also the first death due to the virus, albeit in a multi-storey residential complex in Baliga Nagar with good sanitisation facility and scope for social distancing. But alarm bells rang 4 days later when the virus found its way to one of the largest and most dense slum clusters, Mukund Nagar. Controlling the spread of infection in an area where 5 to 10 people stay in a 10×10 square feet room, was seen as almost impossible. The MCGM swung into action: within 48 hours, it barricaded the entrance and exit to the slum cluster, carried out disinfection of 425 public toilets, began door-to-door screening, and provided food to people in the first month of the world's strictest lockdown to slow down the spread of the pandemic. From roping in private and local medical practitioners to classifying every Covid-19 contact as "high risk", given the density in the Dharavi slums, the MCGM took bold and smart calls over the last 2 months.'

Bhalerao was impressed enough to add in her report: 'In due

[4] *The Indian Express*, 21 June 2020.

course, the MCGM brought in private practitioners to create an environment of trust for people to come out and report symptoms. fever camps were set up to isolate vulnerable people and shift high-risk contacts from slums to institutional quarantine. The civic body also took over some private hospitals, so that it had adequate treatment capacity. Against a 5-day compounded daily growth rate (CDGR) of almost 23 per cent on 20 April, Dharavi's 5-day CDGR on 20 June dropped to 0.85 per cent.

'In fact, a steady decline in cases has prompted the MCGM to consider an "unlock" plan for Dharavi. This may include opening of small-scale industries, and pottery work with minimum staff. The focus of the civic body is now restricted to just four hotspots—Matunga Labour Camp, 90 Feet Road (Sai Baba Nagar), Dharavi Cross Road and Kunchi Korve Nagar—which are still showing a rise in cases. The total number of Covid-19 cases in Dharavi stands at 2,158. Its daily growth rate is 1.57 per cent compared with the city's 3 per cent. While there were no deaths recorded between 30 May and 8 June, 7 deaths have been reported since, taking the total toll in Dharavi to 79.'

The optimism would last through the next 8 months up to February 2021 when a vicious second wave struck Mumbai and then the rest of India. Dharavi was not spared. But the measures already in place ensured that the impossibly congested slum would suffer less than could be rationally expected.

Chahal says the civic body's work in Dharavi was quick to attract global attention. The BBC's Soutik Biswas, addressing a global audience, lauded the success of Dharavi in containing the virus, but entered a note of caution at the end of his report:[5] 'Imagine more than 6,50,000 people spread over 2.5 square kilometres, less than a square mile. That's a population larger than Manchester living in an area smaller than Hyde Park and Kensington Gardens. 8 to 10 people live together

[5]BBC, 22 June 2020.

in poky 100 square feet dwellings.

'About 80 per cent of the residents use community toilets. Homes and factories coexist in single buildings lining the slum's narrow lanes. Most people are informal daily-wage workers who don't cook at home and go out to get their food.

'And yet Dharavi, a sprawling slum in the heart of Mumbai, India's financial and entertainment capital, appears to have brought an outbreak under control—for now. The scale of the measures put in place—a mix of draconian containment, extensive screening and providing free food to an out-of-work population—has been extraordinary. Municipal officials say they have traced, tracked, tested and isolated aggressively to halt the spread of infection. At the heart of this has been the screening effort, involving fever camps, doorstep initiatives and mobile vans. The early door-to-door screening by workers in sweltering personal protective gear was not sustainable when the weather turned hot and muggy.

'Private doctors have joined the fever camps. The cash-rich municipality, politicians, and non-profits have provided tens of thousands of free meals and rations. Bollywood actors and businessmen have donated gear, oxygen cylinders, gloves, masks, medicines and ventilators. "Mumbai has a history of community action. They have done a good job in helping officials contain the infection in Dharavi," says Dr Armida Fernandez, who's involved with a non-profit working in the slum.

'The slum is home to thriving leather, pottery and textile stitching businesses. It has 5,000 small factories which pay taxes. It is also Mumbai's main hub of plastic recycling. Not surprisingly, Dharavi is a place where migrant low-cost skilled labour has thrived for decades. After the lockdown, an estimated 1,50,000 of them left the place for their native villages after their workplaces shut and their earnings dried up. Residents have pawned their gold, depleted their savings and been pushed into debt.

'Questions remain. Will there be enough water in a slum where many buy supplies to make sure that people can wash their hands? Will there be enough jobs left to woo workers back to the factories? How long can the slum remain in a lockdown mode to contain future waves of infection? How long can non-profits continue to help as they start to run out of resources in what promises to be a long and weary battle?'

The answers would arrive months later. In both the first and second waves of the pandemic, right through to the start of 2022, Dharavi served as a microcosm of how the "Mumbai Model' could be replicated to successfully overcome the Covid-19 pandemic.

The Union government, often at odds with the MVA government in Maharashtra, was impressed. As the *Times of India* noted on 21 June 2020: 'The centre praised the Mumbai civic body for actively chasing the novel coronavirus in Dharavi, saying proactive measures reduced the growth rate of the infection in Asia's largest slum to 1.02 per cent in June from 12 per cent in April. The health ministry also lauded the MCGM for ensuring a steep decline of daily Covid-19 cases in Dharavi from an average of 43 in May to 19 in the third week of June. As parts of these efforts, they have actively chased the virus and aggressively conducted targeted tracing of Covid suspects, the ministry said.

'Being densely populated, the civic body faced several challenges in Dharavi where 80 per cent of the population depends on community toilets. The MCGM adopted a model of actively following the four T's—tracing, tracking, testing and treating, the ministry said. This approach included activities like proactive screening. While 47,500 people were covered by doctors and private clinics in house-to-house screening, about 14,970 people were screened with the help of mobile vans, and 4,76,775 were surveyed by municipal workers.

'Fever clinics were set up for screening high-risk categories such as elderly citizens. This helped to screen 3.6 lakh people. Also, around 8,246 senior citizens were surveyed and as part of its policy of "timely separation", they were separated from the other community members to effectively limit the transmission of the disease, the ministry noted. A salient feature of the MCGM's Covid-19 response strategy is strict enforcement of containment measures, which has three primary components—an effective containment strategy, conducting comprehensive testing, and ensuring an uninterrupted supply of goods and essential supplies to the community. Only critical patients were moved outside Dharavi for admission to hospitals and 90 per cent of the patients were treated inside Dharavi itself, the ministry said.

'The MCGM also distributed more than 25,000 grocery kits and more than 21,000 food packets for lunch and dinner separately within the containment zones so that people stayed inside and did not have the need to move out, thereby curbing the spread of the virus. Food and grocery were also supplied and distributed free of cost by local MLAs, MPs, and corporators, the ministry said, adding that there was frequent disinfection of the containment area and community toilets. Maharashtra State Road Transport Corporation buses were operated for facilitating staff conveyance, while the high-risk zone was sealed from all sides and community leaders were appointed as "Covid warriors" to address all issues of the community and to act as a bridge between health workers and the community. This helped to allay any fears and concerns they may have, and bolstered their confidence in the government's efforts, the union ministry acknowledged.'

Chahal adds that the World Health Organization was not only fulsome in its praise for the work done by the civic body in Dharavi to fight the virus, but at made its appreciation plain in public. WHO Director-General Dr Tedros Ghebreyesus said on 11 July 2020 at a press briefing: 'Today, the world recorded 12 million cases. In the last 6 weeks, cases have more than doubled. (But) there are many examples from around the world that have shown that even if the outbreak is very intense, it can still be brought back under control. And some of these examples are Italy, Spain and South Korea, and even in Dharavi—a densely packed area in the megacity of Mumbai—a strong focus on community engagement and the basics of testing, tracing, isolating and treating all those that are sick is key to breaking the chains of transmission and suppressing the virus.'

The World Bank joined the chorus of praise for Dharavi. In its biennial report, *Poverty and Shared Prosperity*, it said that reported cases in Dharavi had been cut to 20 per cent of their peak between May and July. The World Bank pointed out that Mumbai's officials controlled the spread of Covid-19 in Dharavi by involving community members and paramedics. This led to a dramatic fall in both Covid-positive cases and fatalities. It was a lesson, the institution said, that cities across the world could draw from.

On 16 May, 8 days after he took over as municipal commissioner, Chahal convened a meeting of 35 major private hospitals in the city. The meeting with the heads of Mumbai's leading private hospitals took place in the sprawling conference room on the second floor of the MCGM's heritage headquarters. Chahal recalls: 'That day I had a news clipping in my hand from *The New York Times*. I made a very emotional appeal to the CEOs of these private hospitals. I told them that I had been in Mumbai since the last 30 years. I have been reading how medical professionals like you want to make Mumbai the medical tourism hub of Asia. Whenever I have been to a hospital, I have seen foreign patients from the Middle East, Africa and elsewhere sitting in your waiting rooms. You proudly claim that Mumbai is going to be the medical tourism hub of Asia. Then I read out to them the *New York Times* article. It said that Mumbai's health infrastructure had collapsed. The people of Mumbai are going to die like rats. The slums in Mumbai are on fire and totally out of control. Covid-19 is spreading like wildfire. I told the hospital CEOs that our reputation is at stake. People are actually dying on the streets. This is going to get worse.

'By tomorrow you will have 30-40 deaths on the streets of Mumbai and the world is watching. I told them that this pandemic will one day go away. But it will kill thousands of people before that, we don't know how many. But your reputation will definitely take a big hit. Your hospitals' reputation will be gone for the next 20 years and all your plans of making Mumbai a medical hub will go for a toss—unless we join hands and protect our people. The *New York Times* is saying that this is only the beginning of the problem, that Mumbai's health infrastructure is so weak that it is already collapsing with the onset of the Covid-19 pandemic. When Covid-19 is in full virulence with deadly future waves, more and more people in Mumbai are going to die.'

Chahal looks into the distance as he recalls the events of nearly 2 years ago: 'All the private hospital CEOs asked me, one by one, what we wanted from them. I asked them how many Covid beds and ICU beds they could create. Moreover, they had to separate their hospitals into two wings: a Covid zone and a non-Covid zone. The CEOs said they had 4,000 Covid beds and 417 Covid ICUs. I told them to give me control of the 417 ICUs immediately and I will do the bookings there. As far as the 4,000 Covid beds were concerned, I applied the 80:20 formula. I told them to hand over 80 per cent of their beds to the MCGM on a single dashboard and for these we will charge patients our common rates: ₹4,000 for a normal Covid bed, ₹7,500 for an oxygen bed, and ₹9,000 for a ventilator bed.

'I left the balance 20 per cent beds to the private hospitals. They could charge whatever they felt was appropriate for those beds. The MCGM would not ask them any questions. But 80 per cent of the beds in these posh private hospitals would go to slum dwellers. If a rich man is admitted in your 20 per cent quota, I told them, they will go to the same ICU, lie next to each other, and the same doctors will treat the rich and poor patients equally. My patient will pay ₹4,000 per bed per day through the MCGM's grant and your patient can pay you ₹4 lakh per bed per day or whatever he can afford. But both will get exactly the same treatment.'

Subsequent meetings were held on 18 May and 20 2020. All the hospitals unanimously agreed to Chahal's emotional appeal and, the very next day, conveyed their verbal concurrence. The principal secretary to the Maharashtra government issued a notification on 21 May 2020 under the following Acts:

1. The Epidemic Diseases Act, 1897
2. The Disaster Management Act, 2005
3. The Maharashtra Essential Service Maintenance (Amendment) Act, 2011
4. The Maharashtra Nursing Home (Amendment) Act 2006
5. Bombay Public Trust Act, 1950 'B.P.T. Act.'
6. Public Health Department Notification No. CORONA-2020/ C.R.97/Aro-5 Dated 30 April 2020

The notification, with detailed annexures, went on to cap the prices that private hospitals could charge patients. The notification formalised the discussion Chahal had with the CEOs of 35 private hospitals, giving it a legal foundation. 'This proved to be a game-changing initiative,' he says. 'This is unique to Mumbai where hospitals do not allot their own beds. The allotment is done by the MCGM ward war rooms at government rates.'

Chahal quickly put this bed allocation system on an online dashboard. Till then hospital beds were being allotted physically. 'By the end of May 2020,' Chahal notes, 'we had 148 hospitals online, including the 35 major private hospitals, government and MCGM hospitals and smaller nursing homes. I have data on my phone with real-time information on which hospitals have how many vacant beds and what is their exact status. I told every ward officer to create a quota of 100 beds. By 24 May we issued orders with the consent of the private hospitals. By the end of May, bed availability went up from 3,000 to 10,000, apart from Jumbo field hospitals which by then were also under construction. By 15 June the bed count rose to 15,000 and by the end of June, it went up to 22,000 beds. Thus, at the peak of the first wave of the Covid-19 pandemic, we had an inventory of 22,000 available beds, with operation theaters, ventilators, oxygen and ICUs.

'Currently, 144 private hospitals have joined in on a single, real-time, online integrated bed allotment dashboard of the MCGM comprising 30,000 beds, including 3,000 ICU beds in 186 Covid hospitals and 44 municipal government-owned hospitals.'

As the first wave gathered force, Chahal issued an order on 10 June 2020: 'I, I.S. Chahal, Municipal Commisioner, as an empowered officer under provisions of the Epidemic Diseases Act 1897, appoint Dr Gautam Bhansali, Consulting Cardiologist, Bombay Hospital, as Chief Coordinator between MCGM and Private Hospitals for ensuring smooth Hospital Bed Management.

'The Chief Coordinator, as stated above, shall personally contact all the concerned hospitals to coordinate all issues related to his work mentioned above and ensure that maximum patients get seamless and efficient services from all concerned hospitals. He shall remain in contact with the Director, Disaster Management Department of the MCGM, IAS officers appointed to supervise various issues pertaining to the Private Hospitals and report to the undersigned as and when required.

'The appointment as mentioned above is honorary and with the consent of Dr Gautam Bhansali and shall continue till further orders in this regard.'

Along with other senior doctors, Dr Bhansali would play a critical role in the long and difficult battle that lay ahead. Chahal allows emotion to infuse his thoughts: 'The last global pandemic was the Spanish Flu in 1918-20,' he says. 'This pandemic came after 100 years. It gave me an opportunity to help protect the lives of the 15 million people of Mumbai within my jurisdiction. Mumbai is the most complicated city in the world with slums and a high density of people. I am a God-fearing person. I said to myself that there can't be a bigger service to humanity than this enormous responsibility. I made a promise to myself when I spent those 53 minutes in Nair Hospital's Covid ICU ward that I was going to do everything I could. I prepared myself for the worst. There are 5,000 IAS officers in India. I haven't come across a single instance where an IAS officer in the country has put on a PPE kit and entered a Covid ICU ward. It's a deadly place; it's like a death warrant. Every breath you take in a Covid ICU ward can infect you with the coronavirus. The 7 deputy municipal commissioners also never entered Covid ICUs—and rightly so. Why should anyone risk their lives unnecessarily? I entered 3 Covid ICUs: in Nair, KEM and Sion Hospitals and have survived to tell this tale.'

TWO

THE WAR ROOM STRATEGY

Chahal credits his fortitude during the long battle with Covid-19 to a disciplined army background. His father, Lt. Colonel Man Singh Chahal (Retd.), served the Indian Army with distinction. Chahal was born in Sri Ganganagar, Rajasthan on 20 January 1966. An important, if quiet, influence on his early life was his mother Gurdev Kaur. Young Chahal studied at Our Lady of Fatima Convent School, Patiala, and St. Joseph's Convent High School in Pathankot. After completing his 10+2 from Air Force Central School, Jodhpur, Chahal enrolled into the prestigious Thapar Institute of Engineering and Technology (a deemed university), Patiala, and earned a B.Tech (Honours) degree in electronics and electrical communication engineering. Chahal became one of the country's youngest IAS officers in 1989. He is married to Avneet whose father, Ajit Singh Chatha, a senior IAS officer, was the chief secretary of Punjab.

A devoted family man, Chahal has spent much of his career in the IAS in Mumbai and Maharashtra. A fitness aficionado, Chahal has run in every half-marathon held in Mumbai since 2004. Despite his professional and personal accomplishments, Chahal remains grounded. That has helped him cope with the severe challenge of leading Mumbai's fight against Covid-19. It has also brought him global recognition.

In July 2021, as the second wave of the pandemic abated, Chahal was invited to address the European Business Group (EBG) comprising ambassadors and consul generals from Europe. Introducing him to the assembled guests by video conference, the organisers ran through Chahal's career record: district magistrate in the districts of Thane and Aurangabad; principal secretary, urban development; principal secretary, water resources; secretary, medical education; and commissioner, excise department. At the Centre, Chahal has been joint secretary UT, an important charge in the ministry of home affairs and the ministries of women and child development and panchayati raj.

None of these assignments quite prepared him for the challenge Covid-19 posed to the city he had served for 3 decades. Chahal reflects sombrely on the problems Mumbai faced in the initial days of the pandemic: 'The biggest challenge I confronted when I took charge on 8 May was the total chaos in the allotment of beds for Covid-positive patients. Like the rest of the country, the initial system adopted by the MCGM was clear: every evening labs tested people. We had more than 400 flu clinics functioning in April 2020. The flu samples would go to the lab. Once the lab found a Covid-positive test result among the samples, the lab had to do two things.

'First, they had to upload details of the Covid-positive patient on the national portal of the Indian Council of Medical Research (ICMR). That is how the Union government received complete information on how many people were Covid-positive, how many were cured, and how many had died. It is a very comprehensive ICMR medical portal. All tests conducted on a Covid-patient needed to be uploaded on the portal. Second, these labs had to send an email to the concerned patient. The mail would include details of when the sample was taken, the patient's mobile phone number and other relevant information.'

This system ensured that doctors, hospitals, patients and the MCGM were fully briefed. Action, where necessary, could be coordinated seamlessly and quickly. The protocol was in place from March 2020 across the country. It had been prescribed by the ICMR with clear guidelines. Chahal decided to overhaul this protocol for Mumbai. He faced hurdles and criticism but stood his ground.

'Mumbai is the only city in India, and possibly in the world, which adopted this new system,' says Chahal. 'Till today, there is no other parallel. The problem with the exising protocol at the time was that the labs were sending test result messages after 7.00 pm. They would do testing the whole day. Then before closing at around 8.30-9.00 pm, they would send the required mail with the test result and go home. Now people would receive an email at 7.00 pm or later stating that they were Covid-positive. In those days the mortality rate was at 8 per cent. There was no medication and obviously no vaccine. So the first thought that came to your mind when you received a Covid-positive report was that you could die. There was widespread panic about the disease.

'The fear among the patients was palpable. Unless he got a good hospital and was allotted a good bed, he felt his life was in danger. He would use all his resources to get a hospital bed because for him it was a matter of life and death. We had numerous cases of VIPs ringing up their minister friends, IAS officers, trustees of hospitals, top doctors and media barons, requesting them to arrange a good hospital and Covid bed. Each patient generated about 10-12 phone calls. We were getting around 1,700 Covid-positive patients every evening. These 1,700 Covid patients prompted thousands of phone calls every day. During the national lockdown, as per government instructions, every district and every city like Delhi, Mumbai and Chennai had established a central control room for Covid so that if a person became Covid-positive, he could be guided and helped. The helpline number for Mumbai was 1916. So the patient would either ring up that number or someone on behalf of the patient would ring up.'

Chahal pauses to collect his thoughts. 'Now this control room had only 30 MTNL lines,' he says. 'So when hundreds and often thousands of phone calls started coming in every evening between, say, 7.15 pm and 10.00 pm, the system collapsed. The media was keeping a very close watch. These MTNL lines got jammed every evening. The media also rang up these telephone lines to check whether or not they were functioning. This made the situation worse. Television channels, on noting that the MTNL Covid helpline was jammed or constantly busy, started reporting on air at around 8.00-8.30 pm that the Covid helpline had collapsed. This created total panic in the minds of already anxious patients. Those who were healthy were also worried: if tomorrow they too were infected with Covid, they could face the same predicament. The government of India was taking Covid very seriously. Prime Minister Narendra Modi is very focused and always hands-on. I admire him for this. He gets things done by personally monitoring them. The PMO is proactive as well. But this was a peculiar problem.'

Meanwhile, the Union home minister's office was also monitoring the Covid pandemic along with the Union health ministry and the cabinet secretary. They had started receiving calls from influential people in Mumbai. Says Chahal: 'Some powerful person in Delhi—for example, a retired chief secretary or a retired cabinet secretary—would not mind picking up the phone and calling the authorities here regarding the "chaotic" situation in Mumbai. Many times their relatives in Mumbai could not get a hospital bed. They would start ringing them up in Delhi to 'please organise something'.

'After I took over as commissioner, all the single-point phone calls would come to me, whether it was the home secretary or the health secretary or the PMO. All would complain that the helpline is not working, the system is jammed, and no Covid hospital beds are available in Mumbai, something needs to be done. All this would happen between 9.00-9.30 pm to 10.00 pm and go on till past midnight. If I was at dinner and didn't pick up the phone for 10-15 minutes, the VIPs would start phoning the chief minister directly. The CM would call me and say that such and such minister from Delhi has called up, or media channels have called, he is not getting a bed or some relative of his is not getting a bed, what is the current situation, Chahal?

'This was a horrific situation, repeated every evening. First of all, it created a bad impression that the system had absolutely collapsed in Mumbai. Secondly, it created a lot of stress in my mind that I was not able to deliver. Thirdly, it created stress in the minds of the patients. Overall, it painted a very bad picture of the city. Newspapers the next morning would report that many Covid-positive patients did not get hospital beds or medical treatment and because of this several had died. Some politicians even said that the MCGM is helpless, the city has collapsed, the army should be brought in.'

A worried Chahal immediately called a meeting with his core team. These comprised additional commissioners, deputy commissioners, control room staff and senior doctors. Chahal asked them about the series of problems they were facing and what they suggested should be done about them. 'The situation in Mumbai was grim; it couldn't be allowed to go on forever,' the usually unflappable Chahal told the assembled officers. 'If a Covid-positive patient did not get a bed and his oxygen levels fell to 60-65, he could very well die. The family would blame the authorities, accusing the MCGM of carelessness or even callousness.'

As the Covid crisis in Mumbai and across India mounted, senior doctors pointed out that Covid-positive lists were arriving in the evening at a time when healthcare professionals who have to admit these patients in hospitals were fatigued after a long exhausting day on their feet in claustrophobic PPE kits.

'The doctors and healthcare professionals work non-stop from 9.00 am to 7.00 pm,' says Chahal. 'By the time the hospital dean and the senior doctors prepared to leave for home from 7.00 pm onwards, they started getting incessant phone calls. Patients called them. We also called them. They were so fatigued that they were not fully functional at that time. Another perennial problem, the doctors pointed out, was that while we had only 30 MTNL lines, we received over 1,000 phone calls every day. These were the two main reasons they cited for the practical problems they faced. One of my officers, Mahesh Narvekar, who is a deputy commissioner and in charge of the control room, had meanwhile written to MTNL to double the lines from 30 to 60 so that we would get some relief. But I asked him how an additional 30 lines would take care of thousands of cases and calls every day? It was not possible. I told him to forget what the ICMR says or what the labs are doing. We will have to completely overhaul the control room system and protocol. We have to deliver as human lives are involved.'

An animated Chahal recalls: 'People were dying all around us. We used to record 80-100 deaths per day in the first wave. We had to save lives and for that I was ready to go to any extent. Dr Gautam Bhansali of Bombay Hospital, the chief coordinator between the MCGM and the private hospitals, was liaising with hospital managements on our behalf along with his own medical team. I then suggested to Dr Bhansali and the other team members that we should abolish the control room. Some colleagues were taken aback. They said that while the control room may not be working efficiently, if we abolish it completely, what will happen to the city?'

Chahal responded that the problem of an ineffective control room, and its inability to reach out to people, was never going to get sorted out. 'It's terrible that online systems are not available,' he told the assembled doctors, medical staff and others. 'Even if one caller gets through to the helpline with great luck, there is no computer there or even an online mechanism. The person at the other end of the line in the control room says he will call up the hospital to find out about the bed situation. He would call a private hospital and the hospital clerk would tell him that there was no bed available. So then he, in time, would call the patient and inform him accordingly. I pointed out to the doctors at the meeting that we had no inventory: how many beds are occupied, how many we can allot. There simply was no data available.'

From this conversation sprang the game-changing idea of establishing 24 war rooms. Chahal describes how the new policy germinated: 'I told the doctors and the MCGM staff that I was not going to scrap the current system today evening itself. But this Covid fight will go on for a long time. So we have to create systems that function seamlessly and on a long-term basis. The MCGM has jurisdiction over a population of 15 million people. We have 24 wards in Mumbai. These wards are all well established structures and have been functioning since before Independence.

'Each ward is headed by a senior officer and there are thousands of people working under him. So I suggested: why not create one control room in every ward instead of just one MCGM control room? My team thought that creating a totally new system within a government bureaucracy will take a lifetime. They were reluctant; they believed there would be total chaos in the city. But I insisted: here we have one central control room; let us have 24 control rooms with seamless, real-time information connectivity. We started listing out what was required in a control room. All this went on for 3 days, a total of 20 hours of discussion, each discussion lasting over 6 hours.'

Having grown up in army cantonments, Chahal decided to call the MCGM's 24 new control centres "war rooms".

'We set up 24 war rooms in Mumbai,' he says. 'As long as the war against Covid is on, these war rooms will function. I told my team to list out the requirements for each war room. I told them it was my job to arrange the resources needed. I had already decided to get

IIT Bombay and an IT company on board to make, along with our in-house experts, an online dashboard which would flash the live status on everyone's mobile phone: details on each hospital, how many beds were available, how many oxygen beds, normal beds, ventilator beds, how many were occupied, how many were vacant. This system was in existence nowhere else in the country. The Centre had left it to the states.

'We decided to install an online dashboard in every war room. We assigned 10 doctors to each war room. Each dashboard was to be managed by the doctors in 3 shifts. That meant 240 doctors per shift across the 24 war rooms and a total of 720 doctors in 3 shifts. Another 10 per cent would be needed if some doctors fell sick. We would therefore need 800 doctors. At the same time, we had to create 30 telephone lines in every ward. We needed 720 lines across the 24 war rooms. We needed one dozen telephone operators per war room, again in 3 shifts, to manage the calls—around 1,000 operators in all. Remember, in May 2020 almost 50,000 municipal school teachers were sitting at home during the national lockdown, getting their full salary. We decided to induct a thousand among them in the 24 war rooms to monitor calls from leaders of the containment zones. Moreover, each war room must have 10 ambulances and 10 medical teams in PPE kits. Each team should have a paramedical compounder, one assistant and one security guard. Each war room must also have the infrastructure to function seamlessly. And the war rooms must be functional in three 24/7 shifts on autopilot.'

All this created huge logistical problems. Chahal and his team worked round the clock. 'Getting municipal teachers was not a problem,' says Chahal. 'We needed 1,000 and there were 15,000 municipal teachers idle during the lockdown. As far as paramedics were concerned, it was not a problem either as we had a number of health workers. The MCGM has over 50,000 health workers and we needed just 720 for 3 shifts across the 24 war rooms. We had 80 ambulances but we requisitioned another 800 in 15 days. Ambulances were present 24/7 at the 24 war rooms. The only challenge was to get 800 doctors. We spent sleepless nights. One day, I received a phone call from the chief minister on the unavailability of hospital beds. Another day, the Union cabinet secretary called regarding the same issue. The pressure was mounting. The problem of a shortage of doctors to run our war rooms seemed intractable.

'One night I just got up and sat on my bed at 2.15 am. I could not sleep at all. I sat up till 4.00 am thinking about what we needed to do next. Around dawn, an idea struck me. I used to be a secretary in the education department running 52 government/private medical colleges in 2011 and 2012. Maharashtra has more than 27 private medical colleges and 25 government medical colleges. Each of these 52 medical colleges has a batch of 200 medical students in their final year who are completing their internship. They have finished 4.5 years of study. They needed to complete 10 months of internship after which they would get their MBBS degrees. So even at this stage they were as good as doctors. These 52 medical colleges thus had 10,000 trained medical human resources available. They were not deployed anywhere as they didn't have medical degrees. But I did not need their degrees for them to speak to Covid patients from our war rooms and make sure all was well. They were available from all over Maharashtra and even in tribal areas. They were young boys and girls about to get their MBBS degrees but they were all sitting idle during the lockdown.'

When Chahal came to office the next day, he immediately rang up the then dean of Nair Hospital, Dr Mohan Joshi. He told him that he required 1,000 doctors. 'I then called Dr T.P. Lahane,' says Chahal. 'He is a world-famous eye doctor and was till recently the director of Medical Education and Research, Maharashtra. I asked both Dr Joshi and Dr Lahane how we could recruit 1,000 doctors. I told them we have 10,000 boys and girls about to graduate from medical colleges across the state but they are stuck because of the Covid pandemic in the interiors of Maharashtra. Dr Joshi said he would run a social media campaign on WhatsApp. Dr Lahane added that all the deans of the medical colleges in Maharashtra would be sent messages on various WhatsApp groups and asked to inform their internship students.'

Chahal gave the medical students a lucrative offer. He knew they would not normally travel to Mumbai from the interiors of Maharashtra during the total national lockdown. He therefore told the deans to inform the students that they would get free boarding and lodging in five-star hotels in Mumbai within walking distance from the war rooms. The five-star hotels were anyway vacant in May 2020 with no revenue. Besides free accommodation, the medical students would receive, apart from a monthly stipend of ₹11,000 as per regular government policy for medical interns, an enhanced amount of ₹50,000 per month from the MCGM as a special case. These pre-MBBS students would be assigned work in the 24 air-conditioned war rooms in 8-hour shifts.

Social media messages from Dr Joshi and Dr Lahane went out. Chahal and his team awaited the response. 'We were surprised—in just about 3 days we received replies from 1,100 "doctors" awaiting their final MBBS degrees,' says Chahal. 'Dr Joshi was very positive. He told me not to worry as we will be able to recruit over a thousand medical students. The advantage in the MCGM is that I am the final deciding authority and we have a unified command in the city. Otherwise you have to get government approval for making use of funds. I could implement these ideas as the MCGM is not only the richest civic body in the country, with an annual budget of nearly ₹46,000 crore and reserves of ₹87,000 crore, but it is autonomous and invested with tremendous authority under the Municipal Corporation Act to spend money. This is also partly why the "Mumbai Model", as it has come to be known globally, proved successful—because of the kind of financial and operational autonomy we have. This proved to be a great advantage.'

Within 4 days, between 22 May and 25 May, nearly a thousand young medical students arrived in Mumbai from various parts of Maharashtra. War rooms in the 24 wards across the city were scheduled to be inaugurated on 8 June. 'It took us at least 2 weeks to organise all the resources for the war rooms,' Chahal points out. 'MTNL said they would take a week to install the 720 telephone lines we had requested for the war rooms. Arvind Sawant, who is a Member of Parliament and a former Union minister for heavy industries, was the president of the MTNL union for a number of years. He still has tremendous clout in MTNL. On my request, he personally monitored the issue and we had 720 brand new telephone lines installed within 5 days in the 24 war rooms. The other resources—paramedics, ambulances, medical teams, doctors and monitoring teachers—now fell into place. Physical infrastructure in each ward was created for the war rooms. Besides Dr Mohan Joshi, the dean of Sion Hospital, who trained young doctors, I also groomed them personally on Zoom, especially on how to interact with patients.'

On 8 June—coincidentally exactly 1 month after Chahal took charge as municipal commissioner—the 24 war rooms were inaugurated and operationalised. There was criticism though over Chahal's decision to abolish the single control room and establish 24 separate war rooms—thus decentralising the battle against Covid. Kirit Somaiya, the BJP's former Member of Parliament, called Chahal at 9.30 pm on 27 May. Recalls Chahal: 'He said I was playing with fire and that nowhere else in the country had control rooms been abolished. Every state and city has only one control room each, he said. You are the first commissioner who is doing such a thing! No action will take place in these ward war rooms, people will die on the roads, and your reputation will also be at stake. He said he would come and protest outside the MCGM headquarters if the main control room was abolished.'

Chahal kept his cool. He told Somaiya to give him 15 days time.

'I assured him that I would make the Mumbai Model successful. I was determined to make the new structure work. I would go to any extent to control this pandemic. The hospital beds were the main backbone of the Covid fight. If there were no beds, how could you tackle this huge public health emergency? I assured Somaiya again that in the next 15 days if these war rooms don't function satisfactorily as they are supposed to, then he should personally call me. This phone conversation took place on 27 May. Within 12 days our 24 war rooms were operational and they are functional even today. Their performace has been stellar. Somaiya has never called me back till today.'

The MCGM's multiple war rooms became pivots in the fight against Covid. 'We are the only city in the country where we, in effect, created 24 mini-Mumbais through the 24 war rooms,' says Chahal. 'And each mini-Mumbai was fighting the Covid battle independently. To chase the virus, we created a community leader in every containment zone. The teachers were placed in the war rooms to monitor logistics 24/7. There were six teachers in every shift. They were told to each make at least 20 phone calls every day and get feedback from the community leaders on the ground situation in every containment zone. The feedback was put online and passed down to the relevant ward officer. It included information on food packets not reaching patients, doctors not operating their clinics even after taking their free PPE kits, and toilets not being sanitised as per instructions given. The ward officer, who is like a mini-MCGM commissioner, then sent his team to find out the facts and correct any faults.'

The war rooms were the nerve centre of the escalating battle to chase the virus. Over 20 functions went online in real-time: allotment of hospital beds, number of patients quarantined, oxygen procurement, ventilators, ambulances and every other logistical detail. Smitha Nair described in graphic detail[6] the inner working of one war room: '"Can you tell me again how you are related to the patient?" Sangeeta Patil of the Malpa Dongri municipal school, one of the fifty-odd teachers staffing the Covid-19 war room in Mumbai's K-East ward, repeats herself over the telephone. It is a couple of hours into her shift and Patil, tasked with making follow-up calls to patients in home isolation, has just been informed of a patient's death by his relative. How can that be, she asks a colleague. Only 3 days ago, she had spoken to the 53-year-old Prakash Jagdale. He had no symptoms then, and today he is dead. Patil is visibly shaken.

'Around her, a call centre-like humdrum belies the desperation and panic on the other end of the phone calls. "We do show urgency, but there is a thin line between urgency and panic," said Dr Prachi Jadhav, in-charge of the war room. "We have all been trained to be calm and speak with clarity to the patients and their relatives. Our job is to guide them on next steps." One of the key learnings from the early months of the pandemic for the city's civic body, MCGM, has been that strict triaging of patients is essential to ensure the best use of resources. "Triage" is the process of determining the priority of patients' treatments by the severity of their condition or likelihood of recovery with and without treatment. The primary job of the Covid-19 war rooms, one in each of the 24 wards of Mumbai, is that of triaging.

'Here is how it works: An all-Mumbai MCGM bed tracker dashboard provides real-time updates of bed availability across hospitals and Jumbo Covid facilities under various classifications: patients who are Covid-19-positive, further broken down into those who require oxygen and those who don't; suspected Covid-19 patients, also broken down into those who require oxygen and those who don't; patients needing admission to Intensive Care Units, paediatric ICUs, neonatal ICUs; pregnant women; those needing dialysis, and so on. These categories

[6]*Scroll.in*, 26 April 2021.

are further broken down, facility-wise. Each facility is tasked with updating the numbers in real-time.

'Every day, all 24 war rooms receive an online list of Covid-19-positive people in their respective wards from the MCGM's online single-line list collated from all labs, government and private, that are conducting RT-PCR tests. They also receive calls from people who have Covid-19 symptoms and are still awaiting confirmatory tests or test reports. Health workers doing contact tracing on the ground also feed in data about those showing symptoms.'

Chahal clarifies: 'The MCGM receives all positive RT-PCR reports from 56 labs in Mumbai in a single-line list at midnight. By 7.00 am the list is cleaned up by scores of doctors who sit overnight till the early hours of the morning. At 7.00 am, the software automatically splits this list into 24 parts, based on residential addresses shown on the report. Ward war room doctors call up the patients to announce that they are Covid positive; ambulances carrying medical teams reach the patient's residence; the medical condition of the patient is assessed, a bed allotted on the spot and the patient transported in the same ambulance to the allotted hospital bed.'

This is a concept unique to Mumbai in the world, says Chahal.

> Nair adds in her report: 'The war room staff are primarily municipal school teachers, many of whom come from as far as Palghar, Vasai and Virar, mobilised for Covid-19 duty. They are supported by data entry operators and doctors. The teachers call each person on the list and record all details, including oxygen saturation levels, symptoms, comorbidities, vaccine status and the type of house they live in. The last data point helps in deciding if home isolation is indeed feasible, Jadhav said. The doctors in the war room use this data to begin triaging and liaising with hospitals and Covid-19 facilities within their ward. In case of bed unavailability in the ward, the doctors

> contact other ward war rooms using the information displayed on the dashboard. Ambulances are then dispatched to move the patients for whom the doctors have recommended hospital admission.'

Nair's report goes on to describe the crises that frequently emerge: 'Jadhav has been handling affairs at the war room for K-East ward, which comprises the suburbs of Andheri East, Jogeshwari East, and Vile Parle East, since May last year. To her, the pandemic feels interminable. Many in the team have worked weeks without a break, she said. And while set protocol and processes help to keep things running, the shortage of medical facilities had been felt acutely when cases surged dramatically for a few days in March 2021. On an average, the war room was fielding upto 2,000 calls a day, she said.

'Dr Nilesh Tiwari, entrusted with keeping record of and dealing with airport cases—the Mumbai airport is part of the K-East ward—and ensuring enforcement of the hotel quarantine protocol, said they are keenly aware that sometimes their best effort may not be enough, but the learning curve has been steep and every individual in the war room has stepped up to the challenge. The war room reports to Dr Urmila Patil, the medical officer of health for K-East ward. Patil insists that the 2 MCGM and 6 private hospitals in her jurisdiction have for the most part, been adequate. "But last Sunday we faced a crisis situation at one of the private hospitals," she recalled. 5 patients at the hospital were on BiPAP machines that deliver non-invasive oxygen support, but the hospital started running out of oxygen. "I got a call saying my patients will die if I don't get oxygen."

'Unable to procure oxygen immediately, Patil's team looked for an alternative hospital. "We figured that 7 Hills (an MCGM-run hospital with a 2,000 bed capacity) had oxygen but no vacant (oxygen) beds, so we moved the 5 patients with their BiPAP machines, each one accompanied by the attending nurse, into ambulances and rushed them to 7 Hills and transferred them onto a regular bed," she said. "All 5 are fine now."

"Patil's mobile phone rings incessantly. Before the ward war rooms became operational, it was her number, as the medical officer of health, that was circulated widely. "So everybody, from the commissioner down to the last person in the ward, called on this number," she said, throwing her hands up in mock frustration as the phone rang again. It was a member of the contact tracing team, one of the many across the 12 health posts or Arogya Kendras, calling with feedback. Feedback from team members with on-ground experience, she said, has proved helpful in establishing and tweaking protocol. "We are learning as we go along," she says.'

Mumbai's 24 war rooms became a critical asset for monitoring the slum population. It was impossible to monitor slums from one control room. The war rooms made it possible. Each had access to every bed in the city and real-time access to the dashboard. 'The *New York Times* had predicted that people in Mumbai are going to die like rats,' says Chahal. 'What actually happened in New York under former Governor Andrew Cuomo is well known. We have done remarkably well in comparison. We got beds at Hinduja, Lilavati and Breach Candy Hospitals for ₹4,000 a day; 144 hospitals surrendered their entire institutional control to us based on trust. The hospital trustees told me, we want to help you. These hospitals have lost collectively several thousand crore rupees but they have never complained. I fall short of words to express my gratitude to the private hospitals of Mumbai led by their doctors and trustees. One feature is unique to Mumbai: where else in the world would you have the richest and the poorest patients lying in the same ICU, in the same hospital clothes, being treated by the same doctors, receiving the same care and medicines?'

As the first wave of the Covid-19 pandemic swept through Mumbai,

Chahal recalls: 'Our war room doctors were making five to six phone calls to patients every day, asking them if their symptoms had improved or worsened, if they have a temperature, if they are feeling breathless or whether any other symptoms were showing up. This became a seamless, real-time monitoring system. Nowhere else were asymptomatic patients being taken care of in this manner. These medical students, all just months away from getting an MBBS degree, had come from small towns. They were so proactive and energetic. They were enjoying their work. It was also like training for them. Not even one resigned from his or her duties during those difficult days. A Harvard University professor had a Zoom meeting with our team for 1 hour and 40 minutes. He said nowhere in the world did this kind of system exist to his knowledge. As I told him and the others, these decentralised war rooms performed several functions. They have now also been deployed partly to monitor the vaccination drive. The multiple war room concept is a unique feature in our fight against Covid.'

Meanwhile, there were two other challenges that Mumbai faced. One, to ensure ambulances for every emergency; and two, to receive online information about available beds for every big, small, government, private and MCGM hospital. 'At one point of time we had 146 private hospitals on board,' says Chahal. 'Our dashboard displays availability and non-availability of hospital beds, the number of ICUs available, oxygen beds, ventilator beds, everything is on the dashboard to check in real-time. The biggest challenge was to update this information every half an hour. We put competent employees in each of these municipal hospitals as data entry operators. Their only job was to update the dashboard data every half-hour. We placed two municipal auditors in all private hospitals. We also deputed one IAS officer in every municipal hospital. They were officers of the rank of collector. We have 18 municipal hospitals and 2 government hospitals, JJ Hospital and King George Hospital. We created special war rooms in every big hospital, also monitored by IAS officers.'

The four pillars in Mumbai's Covid fight in the first wave were testing, ambulances, doctors and hospitals. In the vastly more lethal subsequent wave in 2021, the focus shifted to oxygen, vaccination and pre-emption. When Chahal took charge as municipal commissioner, the MCGM had only 80 ambulances for a population of 15 million within the MCGM's jurisdiction.

'When I joined,' Chahal rues, 'a number of politicians and citizens were complaining about the non-availability of ambulances. During the first wave, Mumbai's healthcare infrastructure was woefully inadequate. The chief minister had mentioned in one meeting that Jitendra Awhad, Maharashtra's housing minister, was admitted to Jupiter Hospital. He was put on a ventilator. He was very critical and had to be shifted from Jupiter Hospital in Thane to Fortis Hospital in Mulund. The journey is just half-an-hour long, but for 4 hours an ambulance was simply not available. The CM remarked that if an ambulance is not available for a minister for 4 hours, then what will happen to the common man?

'When I became commissioner, all the complaints regarding ambulances started coming to me. I spoke to my team and we decided to innovate. The team suggested that we could convert mini-buses or BEST buses into ambulances in workshops. If we requisitioned private sector ambulances, then the private hospital system would collapse as they too require ambulances in such a grave public health crisis. I had worked as district collector from 1997 to 2004 and conducted a large number of elections, including the 1999 and 2004 Lok Sabha elections. I had also conducted Vidhan Sabha elections in 1999 and 2004. I told my team to follow the election model.

'The election law says that if I need 2,000 vehicles, trucks, tempos, cars, jeeps, I just have to tell the Regional Transport Office (RTO). Any vehicle can be requisitioned by the RTO. So, we decided to put the RTO on duty and said we would compensate them. I called the state transport commissioner. I told him I need 800 Innovas and Sumos in 3 days. I then called Environment Minister Aaditya Thackeray, requesting him to put in a word. It would make things move faster if he spoke to the transport commissioner of Maharashtra who sits in Bandra (a western Mumbai suburb) in the collector's office. I was grateful to Mumbai's Guardian Minister Aaditya Thackeray who followed up with the transport commissioner. In just 5 days, they made arrangements for 800 vehicles along with drivers. Minister Aaditya Thackeray has been a pillar of strength for me and his maturity level at his age always astonishes me.

'We have our own BEST workshop where 4,000 BEST buses are parked and repaired. I told the workshop staff to put an aluminium partition sheet between the driver seat and the rest of the vehicle in all the Innovas and Sumos that we had requisitioned. A Covid patient does not go into a coma. If he has a temperature, or a bad throat, he can sit in the ambulance and reach the nearest hospital in 20 minutes. A stretcher is not required. We thus got 800 vehicles ready with aluminium partition sheets to segregate the patient from the driver and had "Ambulance" painted on all four sides. I could, however, understand the drivers' mental state. They would be terrified that they could be infected by the virus when they open the ambulance door for the patient. So we decided to put 7 PPE kits—one week's quota—in advance under his seat in each ambulance as an additional precaution for the drivers.

'We distributed several hundred PPE kits to the drivers. When their PPE kits were exhausted, they could collect them from the war rooms in their areas. So the war rooms in turn became distribution centres too. We fixed the drivers' compensation at ₹2,000 a day. During the lockdown, these vehicles were idle, making no money at all. At least now they were able to earn something. They were ready to work for the MCGM. Not even one refused. That's how we increased the number of ambulances from 80 to 826 by 25 May. We also requisitioned 50 mini-buses from BEST and converted them into stretcher ambulances for those patients who were differently abled or too old or too sick to sit up and reach the hospital. In another 15-20 days the mini-bus ambulances too became operational. We now had 130 ambulances with stretchers (including the original 80) and 746 ambulances without stretchers, a total of 876 ambulances. Out of these, 240 ambulances were placed at the 24 war rooms.'

The next step was even more innovative. Chahal explains: 'Uber vehicles were also idling during the lockdown. We called the Uber management and spoke to the CEO. We told him that we did not need his vehicles, drivers or any other assistance from Uber. We only needed their software. I told him that we will pay for the software. It is among the best in the world. They were ready to share the software with us. So our ambulances were put on the Uber platform. These were now Uber ambulances—on call. I mentioned to the cabinet secretary of India that we were on the Uber platform. Everything was free: the patient did not have to pay for the ambulance or the hospital stay. Besides, we had not, contrary to some reports, totally abolished the main control room. We were controling the 24 war rooms from the main control room. The 1916 helpline would ring in the war rooms as well. Over 50 ambulances were parked in the main control room of the MCGM. They were on standby in case a patient does not get an ambulance from his war room for any reason. We could then send one from the main control room.'

The media reacted positively to these moves. 'After 15 June, no politician, no citizen, no media person reported in the print, electronic or digital media regarding a lack of ambulances,' Chahal says. 'The ambulance experiment became a success. It killed a number of birds with one stone. It gave income to vehicle owners and employment to drivers who were jobless, while Uber shared its software and platform with us on a commercial basis. We got 876 ambulances. It was a win-win situation for all.'

The next task was to get a list of Covid-positive patients from the labs. Matching the list with available hospital beds was another challenge. 'I took a serious view at my meetings with the CEOs of these labs,' says Chahal. 'At the time there were just 22 labs. Now there are 56. Each lab has dozens of centres across the city. But there was a major testing problem in these labs. Initially, they were driven by commercial considerations. Some big labs have been operational for many years. They now saw a great opportunity. In those days, one Covid test cost ₹4,500; today it has come down substantially. These labs would bite off more than they could chew. I did a study: for swabs taken on 4 April 2020, the results arrived on 22 April 2020. I came down heavily on the CEOs of these labs. I told them that people were dying all over the city, and for tests done on 4 April the results coming on 22 April was terrible. Many of the people awaiting their test results could have died for lack of interim treatment. I gave them the names of those patients who had done their tests on 4 April and died on 11/12 April. Their Covid-positive reports had come on 22 April. This was a crime.

'Moreover, we now had to tap high-risk contacts. If a person had tested positive, his close relatives, like his wife, children, parents, driver and domestic help, had to be taken care of. But many patients had died because of the labs' greed and the absolute chaos in some labs. I told the CEOs that what they were doing was a crime against humanity. I said I did not care that they were registered, sanctioned and approved by the ICMR. They had to function in our city, they had to obey all our rules. First rule: no lab shall take on more tests than their capacity. Second rule: only take on tests whose results you can process in 24 hours. Third rule: all samples collected during the day should be processed and finished on that day. At the end of the day zero samples should be pending.'

Chahal ordered the labs to post a written document every day:

how many samples were collected that day, how many had been processed, how many disposed of, and how many were still pending with them. The results of the tests had to be filed mandatorily in 24 hours.

'At midnight,' Chahal says, 'they had to give us a list of all the positive and pending cases. At that time the labs were doing 11,000 tests per day. I had told them that even if one sample is pending, they will get a show cause notice. First time, there will be a warning and a penalty. Second time, if I find things are not improving at their end, they will have to shut shop in Mumbai. They can go and complain wherever they want—ICMR, Union government, state government. I would answer them, till them why I shut their shop. I was not stifling them or putting a ceiling on them regarding the number of tests they can process. But whatever they take on, they have to complete within 24 hours. They were free to decide their targets and their capacity of testing. It took me a couple of meetings with the CEOs and around 3 weeks before things fell into place. I also had to suspend the licence of 2 very well-known labs. Both got suspended, first for 15 days and then for 1 month.

'I faced a lot of pressure regarding the suspension of their licence. There were allegations that I wanted to reduce testing to show lesser number of Covid-positive patients. The charge was that Mumbai had no available beds for covid-positive patients. I made it very clear to the labs that at midnight they must give us an online list of Covid-positive patients. At midnight, except the MCGM, nobody in the world would know who is Covid-positive in Mumbai. The confidential mail should come only to us. I had to stop all these thousands of phone calls from the patients, their relatives and VIP contacts coming on a daily basis. But if they don't know who is Covid-positive, how will they call ? If the labs shared this information with anyone else, I would issue them a show cause notice, impose a penalty and then shut their shop. They had to upload the information only on the ICMR portal.

Only we have access to it and the labs have access to it—no one else has access to it till a certain time point.'

The MCGM dashboard has 35 pages and is accessible worldwide. 'It gives you every possible information about the Covid fight in Mumbai,' says Chahal. 'At a glance you know how many people are Covid-positive, asymptomatic, negative, how many tests have been conducted till today, etc. It is available to every news media—online, print and electronic. Commenting on the dashboard, the *Washington Post* wrote that it is the most transparent in terms of real-time data. The newspaper had done a survey of Delhi, Chennai, Kolkata and Mumbai to check Covid numbers. They said Mumbai scores high marks for data transparency. Other information that the dashboard provides is the growth of the virus, ward-wise, new cases and deaths, again ward-wise.

'Data entry is an important factor. Whatever data you read in the newspapers every morning is all taken from our website's dashboard. The dashboard reassures citizens that we are not hiding anything. Otherwise, in many other geographies, you get fudged reports on the number of positive patients, on the number of deaths and so forth. On our dashboard, everything is available in the public domain. This dashboard has been useful to health professionals and citizens alike.'

Recounting how the long battle to subdue the first wave of the pandemic was fought—and won—Chahal says: 'This virus is very peculiar in that it spreads like wildfire. Infectivity is very high. June, July and August 2020 were the months when we witnessed the peak of the pandemic's first wave. Luckily, our infrastructure was in place. So we effectively fought the war against the first infectious wave from July to October 2020. We countered the second wave between February-November 2021 and prepared for a third wave towards the end of 2021. If we had not established automated systems and picked up people from the slums, they would have created several new waves. Delhi, for example, had peaks within waves. There is a wave and there is a peak. You can have multiple peaks in a single wave. Here in Mumbai we had one wave and one peak, and then after 10 February 2021, a second lethal wave followed by the Omicron surge in 2022.

'The first peak in the initial wave came roughly around June-August 2020. It settled down gradually. Deaths were maximum in Mumbai in June. It is remarkable how a big metropolitan city which is so complicated in terms of its slum population demographics could avoid a second wave for nearly a year after the first wave of the pandemic had struck Mumbai in February-March 2020. Our systems targeted slums and small tenements. The majority of the work done by our war rooms focused on vulnerable people from slums and shanties. The task was tough: taking care of food packets, sanitisation and comorbid patients. We had to ensure that doctors' clinics remained open, PPE kits were distributed to them, slums cleaned regularly,and health workers monitored closely.'

On 5 June 2020, the MCGM had issued detailed guidelines for testing. It added in a corrigendum on 13 June:

- The laboratory shall intimate all positive status of the patient first to the MCGM and it shall be the duty of the MCGM to further intimate to the patient. The actual copy of the report of the patients can be shared with patients directly but on the subsequent day of intimation to the MCGM ONLY after 11.00 am.
- The information of swabs of high-risk contacts of Covid-positive patients taken at their home premises shall be shared with the ward war room of that ward immediately. The above directives should be implemented forthwith.

Chahal convinced the labs to adhere to this protocol. 'The suspension of the licences of the 2 big labs began at the end of May and went on till 15 July before things actually fell into place,' he says. 'From 5 June to 5 July, all operations of one of Mumbai's biggest labs were shut down. They complained all over. But I did not budge. One of our state ministers called me, saying testing was going down and the suspended lab should be allowed to test. I told him that testing did not make sense if they gave the reports after 8 to 10 days. Once the new protocol was established, we would get the online list by midnight. We had an SOP in place.

'We had one shift of doctors, microbiologists and our own people in the epidemic cell who functioned from midnight to 8.00 am. They were told that when the online list from the labs arrives, they must clean up the list. There were a number of issues involved in this cleaning. Sometimes, the labs sent incorrect addresses. Those patients' names which did not fall into the MCGM's geographical jurisdiction under the larger Mumbai Metropolitan Region (MMR) had to be segregated and transferred to the relevant municipal corporations (Thane, Kalyan, etc.) through the night.

'This was the first part of cleaning the list. Second, we had to check whether a particular patient was a discharge case or an admission case. In those early days when a patient was admitted to a hospital, he would undergo another Covid test. He may continue to be positive and remain hospitalised. So we would have to allot a bed to him again. On our online system, we had created a protocol to clean all such duplicates. This operation would go on from midnight till 6.00 am. The online system would, at 7.00 am, with a single click, split into 24 parts automatically with addresses for action by the 24 war rooms. Now at one minute past seven, for doctors sitting in, for example, the K-west ward, encompassing the Juhu Lokhandwala area, 8 patient names per dashboard would appear. Then at 8.00 am sharp, the first phone call would be made.

'We had trained our people on how to inform the patients that they were Covid-positive. We trained the young staff on duty to say good morning, that he or she was from such and such war room of a particular ward. Then they were to gently inform the persons tested that they were Covid-positive, ask the patient how they were feeling and tell them not to worry at all, that we had plenty of beds available in hospitals. The Covid-positive person would give three or four types of answers about having a temperature or a bad throat or breathlessness or maybe no symptoms at all and they could be feeling fine. If they would say that the symptoms are not showing, then the medical students in our war room would ask them if they would like to be home-quarantined or go to a hospital. If the person preferred to be home-quarantined, then we would inform them that if they develop any symptoms in the next 7 days, they should immediately inform us on such and such number and we will be in touch with you. In case they wanted any guidance regarding Covid, we would connect them to different doctors.'

What if an asymptomatic person had tested positive but was living in a slum and did not have a separate bathroom or a spare room to quarantine himself in? Chahal replies: 'The war room staff would in such a case tell him that an ambulance was being sent for him. He would, be shifted to a Covid Care Centre for asymptomatic people who did not have an independent toilet and bedroom in their house. If their symptoms increased, they would be sent to a Covid hospital. If they didn't have symptoms, they would be tested on the seventh day and the fourteenth day. If they tested negative, they would be discharged.'

Chahal drew a sharp distinction between the behaviour of patients from slums and those from high-rise buildings. In an interview with Shekhar Gupta, founder-editor of the news portal *The Print,* Chahal said: 'During the first wave, from March to December 2020, the majority of patients, around 95 per cent, were from the slums. They were very disciplined, they would never force the lab to share their test report, they would wait for the ambulance to come and pick them up, wait for the phone call to be made by the doctor. They were happy that following a swab taken at 2.00 pm, they would get a phone call the next morning by 8.00 am regarding their status. And again by 2.00 pm they would be on a hospital bed if needed. In the second wave, 95 per cent of all patients came from non-slum areas. Only 5 per cent came from slums.'

As Covid-positive cases rose across Mumbai, an increasing number of patients needed ventilators or oxygen beds. Many had developed a bad throat or a cough and cold. These could develop into a more serious infection. The young medicos manning the 24 war rooms told them not to worry, the medical team, geographically segregated, would come in PPE kits, in an ambulance, and pick them up in the next 20 minutes. The medical team would arrive with the ambulance at the stated time and check the infected person. They first monitored his oxygen level and took his temperature. They carried mobile x-ray sets and took chest x-rays. They showed the results immediately: whether oxygen levels were normal, temperature was fine and chest clear.

Chahal accessed all this information and data in real-time. 'If the person was infected, he was given a choice of going to a government hospital or a private hospital either in north Mumbai or south Mumbai,' he explains. 'After this, the medical team did not immediately leave the person's house. They first called up the specified war room and checked for the availability of beds in the hospital of the person's choice. If a bed was not available in that particular hospital, they offered the patient other hospitals. Availability of beds was checked in several hospitals and a bed number allotted to the person. The patient was then informed, for example, that he had been allotted oxygen bed number 45 in Breach Candy Hospital. The medical team waited for the person to get ready, took him in the ambulance and dropped him to the hospital bed. Once the patient was placed on the allotted hospital bed, the medical team called the war room to confirm that the patient had been taken care of and was on his designated bed. As soon as our medical team entered the hospital, the entire system came under our control. No one could stop them from placing the patient on the specific bed allocated to him by our online system. If anyone objected, that person could be arrested under the Epidemic Diseases Act 1897.'

The Epidemic Diseases Act, 1897 has wide-ranging powers. The British had promulgated this act to deal with epidemics that were frequent in the nineteenth and early twentieth centuries. It remains on the statute book. The MCGM started operating under this act from 11 March 2020, when the pandemic was still in its nascent stages.

The MCGM's online system on lab test results and hospital bed allocation, meanwhile, proved effective. 'The phone calls became history,' smiles Chahal. 'One electronic media journalist did not fully understand the system. I had gone to the Andheri Sports Complex to inaugurate a zero-mission programme that would reduce Covid cases to zero in wards with a high number of Covid infections. On 24 June, the war rooms had been in operation for 16 days. This TV journalist confronted me the moment I came out of the Andheri Sports Complex. We were live on national TV. She told me she had called up Hinduja Hospital about the non-availability of beds. Patients were running from pillar to post for beds. I told her to withdraw her question. I said that in our decentralised war rooms, from midnight till 8 o'clock in the morning, except us no one else knows who is Covid-positive. So if you don't know your Covid report, how can you ring up the hospitals? I told her that at 8.00 am we call up all the covid-positive patients to inform them that they are infected and that we will be coming to escort them within 20 minutes to the hospital. So what is the need for anyone to call up the hospital? Secondly, we had told all the hospitals that if anyone calls up for beds, they have to call up the MCGM. It is a unified online allotment. Given this system, the journalist should have withdrawn her question. But she just put her live TV feed off! This system, though, became a success. We decided to call it *chase the patient* policy. Right from his lab report to putting the patient on the allotted hospital bed, we chased him. This protocol too, does not exist anywhere else in India or the world.'

The system, however, came under immediate attack. On 19 June 2020, a PIL was filed in the Supreme Court. The writ petition said that the municipal commissioner was violating the right of a patient to get his test report directly. 'Tushar Mehta, India's solicitor general, stated that a patient should directly receive the report,' recalls Chahal. 'When this message came to me in the evening at around 6.00 pm, I was demoralised. I thought my entire online, decentralised 24 war room system is going to collapse. The Supreme Court observed at the hearing of the PIL that the patient must get the reports directly.

'Now what happened was this: the Supreme Court judgement came at 11.00 am on 19 June 2020. Suresh Kakani, our additional commissioner who looks after hospitals, had earlier suggested that once we get the online list of Covid-positive patients in the morning, and once beds are allotted by 1.00 pm, we should tell the labs to email the reports to the patients directly. I had accepted Kakani's very sensible suggestion. I issued the relevant order at 8.00 pm on 18 June 2020. By sheer luck, it was the day before the Supreme Court order. God helps those who are sincere in their efforts.

'I then clarified to Ashish Wad, the permanent counsel of the MCGM in the Supreme Court, that the Supreme Court had not said that patients should get their reports *before* or *after* the MCGM but simply that they should get their reports directly. My 18 June order, issued at 8.00 pm, had stated precisely that.'

Chahal adds: 'We filled an affidavit in the Supreme Court mentioning every detail. The case came up for hearing on 7 July 2020 but we did not face any problem during the hearing. I had told my officers that my conscience was clear. If the Supreme Court had summoned me, I would have appeared. But I refused to dismantle the war rooms or dilute their effectiveness.'

The Maharashtra government was pleased with the success of the Mumbai Model. Chahal acknowledges the support he has received through the pandemic from Chief Minister Uddhav Thackeray: 'I have never come across a CM like Uddhav Balasaheb Thackeray who is not only a thorough gentleman, but also gave me a complete free hand and absolute support. He virtually left everything to me. He is a rare politician who has earned respect but never commanded it, unlike many others. I shall remain indebted to him forever.

'The architect of the MVA government and one of the finest leaders Maharashtra has produced, Sharad Pawar not only kept a close watch on the Covid-19 crisis, but also fearlessly travelled to every nook and corner of the state, depicting time and again that age is only a number. His extraordinary energy levels even put today's youth to shame. He asked me to visit Pune, the new coronavirus hotspot in the country at the time and guide the local administration.'

Chahal went to Pune and Nagpur to advise their municipal corporations. Deputy Chief Minister Ajit Pawar was present at the Pune meeting on 17 July 2020 where Chahal addressed several IAS officers. 'Ajit Pawar had full confidence in my capabilities and always supported me to the core,' says Chahal without mincing words. 'Once, he called me and told me that I was a lucky mascot for the government. "Be careful, *aapko nazar naa lage*", he added emotionally.'

Another state minister accompanied Chahal to Nagpur for a similar meeting on 29 August. Senior doctors from Mumbai were present at the meeting along with locally deputed IAS officers and collectors to discuss how the first wave of the Covid pandemic could be tackled with a combination of technology, tracking, tracing, testing and treatment.

And yet, not everyone was convinced. As the United States and Europe grappled with high fatalities, India's low death numbers had first raised questions in the international media as early as July 2020.

Writing in the *Washington Post*, Joanna Slater and Nina Masih noted[7]: 'India is not the only country with a high number of reported cases and relatively low official fatalities. In an interview with CNN, Kremlin spokesman Dmitry Peskov defended Russia's low death rate. "Have you ever thought about the possibility of Russia's healthcare system being more effective?" Peskov asked. In India, one factor that experts say may indeed be lowering the death toll is its predominantly youthful population. According to the most recent census, only 5 per cent of Indians were 65 or older, while more than half were under age 25. Although much remains unknown about the virus, studies have shown that older people are far more likely to experience severe or fatal outcomes.

'Even in developed countries, the full extent of deaths linked to Covid-19, the disease caused by the novel coronavirus, has not been reflected in official statistics. Instead, experts have attempted to analyse "excess deaths"—the ways in which overall deaths have deviated from prior years—as a proxy for the impact of the pandemic. The *Washington Post* contacted officials in four of India's largest cities—Mumbai, Delhi, Chennai and Kolkata—to obtain data for total deaths in each month from March to June for 2019 and 2020. Only Mumbai provided full and up-to-date figures. (Kolkata provided none.)

'In Mumbai, the first city in India to be swamped by a wave of coronavirus cases, overall deaths in March were actually lower than those in the same month in 2019. Officials say the decrease was likely due to the strict nationwide lockdown, which reduced deaths from such events as car accidents. In May, however, total deaths in the city surged to 12,963 compared with 6,832 in the same month a

[7]17 July 2020.

year before. The difference is larger than the number of coronavirus deaths registered in the city in May, which was 2,269. Some of the jump is because deaths from prior months—at the height of the lockdown—were registered later, said I.S. Chahal, Mumbai's municipal commissioner. Chahal said the city had also treated many patients from neighbouring areas. Authorities have made efforts to record coronavirus deaths properly, he added, even if it meant that the official death rate increased.

'In June, Chahal ordered hospitals and clinics to register any previously unreported deaths from Covid-19 within the next 48 hours or he would shut them down. The result: More than 800 deaths added to the overall toll. "We've been transparent," Chahal said. "Let other states of India show this courage." In several Indian cities, reports have emerged from graveyards and crematoriums where staff say they are handling more confirmed and suspected deaths from Covid-19 than the official figures reflect. In the city of Vadodara in western India, the official figures show that the total number of coronavirus cases has increased since the start of June. But the number of deaths has barely budged. Some experts say that even while acknowledging the deficiencies in India's data, they're struck by the way its relatively low deaths per million is shared by other countries in South Asia and Southeast Asia, including Pakistan and Bangladesh. "One can always say that this country or that country is fudging its data, but all countries cannot be fudging data at the same time," said Shahid Jameel, a virologist and former chief executive of the DBT/Welcome Trust India Alliance, a public health foundation. He hopes to see further research into whether different populations have divergent immune responses to the virus.'

Chahal was concerned about under-reported Covid-19 fatalities. He recalls one grim moment in particular: 'One day on 6 June, during the first wave, I was examining death figures. Somaya Hospital reported 17 deaths that day. Now how can 17 people die in one day in the

ICU when the ICU itself has a bed capacity of only 20? I asked our deputy commissioner Suresh Kakani to check. He came back saying that these people have not died yesterday, they have died collectively since March-April-May 2020. There had been no proper reporting of fatalities. I went to the chief minister and told him that we had two options: either we keep quiet about this or be bold and transparent with our data. He said, Chahal, be brave and declare everything.

'The next day I issued an order to 147 hospitals to create an entire case file of patients who have died and send it to the epidemic cell of the MCGM. The cell finally certifies deaths and then it goes into the public domain for declaration. Unless these case files come to us, we cannot certify the death of a person. This format is prescribed in the Epidemic Diseases Act, 1897 that governs us in a pandemic. The hospitals were struggling to follow SOPs. There were too many deaths daily. No one had the time to do paperwork. There was lack of knowledge; the epidemic had struck Mumbai after 100 years. Many case papers were not available. Officers had to collect them from different departments. These were the reasons why all deaths were not getting reported.

'I issued an order under the Epidemic Act that all hospitals had 48 hours to come clean. There will be no extension given. After that, if any hospital reports a previous death as a current death, then their licence will be suspended. Initially, the hospitals were very angry. But Kakani called them and explained that if the MCGM does not know of a death then we cannot declare the person dead. Plus the world media will suspect us of hiding the number of deaths—which happened even in New York and other western cities. I issued an order to the war rooms as well to know the number of deaths that had taken place, who had actually died of Covid, who was taken to a hospital and discharged. Our staff went to their respective homes to find out. This was a mammoth operation. We are possibly the only city to carry out such a complex exercise. It took us 6 days to conduct this operation.

'On the morning of 16 June 2020, 862 past unreported deaths were recorded. Our death rate was 2 per cent. Now it suddenly jumped to 6.9 per cent. In May 2020 there had been 220 deaths—almost 70 deaths per day—and all were under-recorded. On the morning of 16 June I wrote a letter to the state government about the 862 deaths which had not been reported. They had either died at home or in transit to a hospital in the period from March to June 2020. The moment we declared the deaths at 1.00 pm on 16 June and the death rate jumped from 2 per cent to nearly 7 per cent, I told my team that all deaths should be reported within 48 hours. Then I issued another order that I wanted daily returns from all the hospitals and nursing homes and that I wanted nil pendency in declaring deaths. From the first week of July 2020, the backlog of reported deaths in Mumbai was over.'

Nationally though, the issue flared up again as the second deadly wave swept across India. On 4 April 2021, the country recorded a high of over 4,12,000 cases. Through April and early May 2021, daily fatalities shot up to more than 4,000. Reports claimed that even these figures were under-reported by a factor varying between two and five times. A full reckoning can be made only when total deaths in the 2 years between January 2020 and December 2021 are matched against an average of total deaths per year in 2014-19. Excess deaths in 2020 and 2021 over the previous 5-year annual average fatalities will provide an indication of the true devastation of the pandemic that emerged, by most rational, science-based accounts, from biolabs like the Wuhan Institute of Virology in China.

For now though, as the second Covid-19 wave engulfed India in mid-2021, floating bodies in the Ganga became grist to journalists' mills, both in India and overseas. Sucheta Dalal, founder-editor of *Money Life,* highlighted the widespread criticism of dead bodies cremated at packed crematoriums during the peak of the second wave. 'The tragic pictures that we saw in many places in India were the long queus at crematoriums and hundreds of burning pyres,' Dalal said. 'But in Mumbai there were fewer deaths, things were under control. Mumbai has 47 crematoriums, when things started getting sticky, Mr Chahal approached IIT Bombay, got them to create a dashboard, put all the crematoriums there, created a helpline and asked people to call up. All the support has been provided by the MCGM. So when people call, they get to know the rush at (a specific) crematorium, get a slot booked and are able to bid farewell to their loved ones. All this is not just by chance, this is preparation, planning this (needs) a war-like approach. But what about the future? Mr Chahal is already working to tackle the third wave of Covid.'

Through the difficult days of the pandemic, human tragedies were heart-rending. Covid-19, especially during the highly infectious second wave in 2021, took countless lives—doctors, journalists, health workers, migrants, MCGM staff, police officers and others. Some stories though ended well. 'At one point, an unknown man sent me an SMS saying that he loved his father very much and his father was dying,' Chahal recalls. 'I could feel his pain as if it were my own father. So I told him to send me his address. It was in a slum. I told the officer in charge of our control room to send an ambulance at that address and bring the patient to KEM, Sion or Nair Hospital. We had given access to the dashboard to all hospital deans so that they could also upload relevant patient data on the dashboard. By 1.00 am the man's father was picked up from the slum and brought to the hospital. After 6 or 7 days, the patient's son messaged me to say that his father had been saved because of us. He was very grateful. Our team had taken care of everything. It is very gratifying, especially when we get the opportunity to save an unknown human life.'

Chahal's eyes cloud over as he says: 'I talk to myself for 15 minutes to half an hour every day. I go over the wrong things and the right things I have done. It inspires one to do more. Boney Kapoor's maid and cook were Covid-positive. So was his daughter Jhanvi Kapoor. He called me through a common friend. Within 7 minutes of speaking to me, an ambulance had reached his house. All three—the cook, maid and Jhanvi—were picked up and admitted to a hospital. In another 30 minutes, a team came to Kapoor's home and sanitised the entire house. Jhanvi Kapoor made a video of the quick and effective treatment she received that saved her life.'

But even as Mumbai fought its way out of the pandemic's first wave, Delhi sank deeper into it. *India Today* compared the trajectory of the virus in the two cities in a searing story titled *A Tale of Two Cities*[8]:

> 'On 25 June, Delhi overtook Mumbai as the worst-affected city in India due to the coronavirus. The reason is simple: Mumbai has controlled the Covid numbers, while the spike in new cases continues unabated in Delhi. Mumbai remained the Covid hotspot for roughly 5 months, but despite its demography, especially with Asia's largest slum Dharavi, it turned out to be a role model in containing the coronavirus.'

Delhi would tame the second wave by July 2021 after suffering from a critical shortage of oxygen that claimed hundreds of lives earlier that summer. But as the first wave of Covid-19 hit Delhi in 2020, the capital city's lack of preparedness and absence of strategy contrasted sharply with Mumbai. *India Today* described as a case study the capital's dire situation in the winter of 2020:

> 'Delhi is still devising ways to control the growing number of cases—the latest being Delhi Chief Minister Arvind Kejriwal's suggestion to impose a partial lockdown in the national capital. The count of active cases in Mumbai is nearly 11,000 while

[8]19 November 2020.

it is approximately 42,000 in Delhi. However, the death toll due to Covid in Delhi is nearly 3,000 more than Mumbai's. So how did Mumbai succeed in getting it right? Why is Delhi struggling? *India Today* compares the two metropolises on key parametres.

'The Maharashtra government remained adamant in the face of pressure by the Opposition and didn't allow the reopening of schools, places of worship, malls, cinema halls, restaurants and local trains. It issued lockdown guidelines instead. Festive gatherings and celebrations were banned. It was perhaps for the first time that Mumbai showed so much restraint during Ganeshotsav. Community Diwali celebrations too were banned. Chhath Puja at beaches was the latest in the long list of activities prohibited to curb the spread of coronavirus.

'*India Today* spoke to three prominent Delhi-based doctors to understand the reasons for the current situation in the city. All three are of the view that the recent spike is due to the festival rush in Delhi markets where neither social distancing norms nor other necessary guidelines were followed by the public at large. Dr Suresh Kumar, medical director of LNJP Hospital, said, "Earlier, there were fewer instances where all members of a family were found positive but these days, we are observing many such cases."

'Similarly, Dr M.C. Mishra, former director, AIIMS, said, "People have celebrated festivals in closed-door environments and that resulted in a higher infection rate. Even one person can infect many in such a scenario because when such parties happen then people don't follow guidelines at all." Dr Girish Tyagi, secretary, Delhi Medical Council, remarked: "We have seen many video clips from Delhi markets where the crowd was maddening and no social distancing was followed. Delhiites are hardly interested in following Covid norms which have been publicised widely by government agencies."

'In Mumbai, people were asked to stay indoors and not more than 5 people could gather in one place. Helpline numbers were issued for passing on information to civic officials. As restrictions eased, face masks were made compulsory and those who flouted rules paid the fine. Dr Gautam Bhansali, consultant physician, Bombay Hospital, says not allowing local trains, schools and malls to open was a big positive step that helped Mumbai. "In a very short span of time, we were able to create large facilities for citizens with private and government hospitals' participation," he adds.

'Doctors and experts also blame the re-opening of public transport in the national capital for rising cases. Delhi Metro and city buses are operating at full capacity, increasing the chances of infection. Mumbai realised early that it had a massive challenge at hand. To control the rising numbers in large slum pockets, especially Dharavi, was not easy. The primary focus of the Maharashtra government was extensive testing. Mumbai was quick to take maximum measures. Multiple teams were formed for door-to-door surveys of different areas. But getting people to cooperate was a challenge as many would not understand the gravity of the situation. Religious heads were then taken into confidence to ensure cooperation and ease the task of ground workers. Numerous fever clinics were set up and many doctors rendered their valuable services day and night in the most dangerous areas even as rising numbers made headlines.'

The report concluded its cases study of the two cities thus: 'MCGM and Mumbai police joined hands and not just informed the masses through drone services about the invisible danger but the police ensured that they stayed away from the sealed zones. Through CCTVs and drone cameras, police kept a hawk-eye on people. Those found positive or developing symptoms were immediately shifted to isolation wards or Covid centres for treatment. Besides, the MCGM realised that several areas did not have proper sanitation facilities and hence, measures for thorough sanitisation of public toilets and cleaning were undertaken. MCGM workers went door-to-door for massive surveys to check on the health of senior citizens. The Delhi government also initiated several campaigns to educate people about the guidelines and appropriate behaviour. Heavy penalties have been imposed on those found violating norms, but somehow (in Delhi) government agencies could not implement the norms strictly (as Mumbai did) during the Navratra and Diwali festivals when large crowds were seen all over the place (in the capital).'

Despite its early success in controlling the pandemic, Mumbai went through its own share of trauma. The paucity of private, government and municipal hospital beds to treat the flood of new Covid-positive patients called for out-of-the-box thinking. The city's battle against Covid-19 was just beginning.

THREE

A JUMBO INNOVATION

Mantralaya, the Maharashtra government's administrative nerve centre, was like a ghost building through the first national lockdown. Fewer than 10 IAS officers and staff attended office to keep the wheels of government machinery moving. An additional problem was looking after the transportation of over 9 lakh migrants workers. They were desperate to return to their hometowns after the national lockdown was partially lifted in May 2020. 'We had to ensure that civil supplies functioned properly during the total national lockdown,' says Chahal. 'Sanjeev Jaiswal, our additional municipal commissioner, was in charge of the movement of groceries, ensuring that bazaars and food outlets continued to function. Other IAS officers looked after relief camps. The state government had opened a large number of relief camps in Maharashtra where migrant labourers were housed. During the March-May national lockdown, everything was shut. There was zero employment, zero work.

'Our immediate concern was this: how would daily wage earners and manual labourers survive? The state government had to plan free meals for them. An IAS officer, Co-operative Department Secretary Abha Shukla, was in charge of every labour camp across Maharashtra. Hundreds of relief camps began functioning.

Several lakh people were accommodated there. We had to take

care of three meals a day for every migrant worker. There was unrest in these relief camps. People needed money in hand for their personal expenses besides food. But there was no work and, especially for daily wage earners, no income.'

The state government announced that it would give ₹2,000 to each migrant worker who was staying in relief camps. 'Every evening and afternoon we would get together at the CM's official residence, Varsha,' says Chahal. 'One day, a covid-positive case got detected in Varsha. We had to put that location also out of bounds. We did not know where to conduct our meetings. In Mantralaya too, a couple of Covid-positive cases arose. The CM decided to hold meetings in the old mayor's bungalow at Shivaji Park, in central Mumbai. The mayor had already shifted to a new bungalow in Byculla and the old one was vacant. This was the state of affairs during the first lethal peak of the pondemic. Around this time, the CM warned us that as Covid-19 spread, we would soon need a large number of hospital beds.'

By now, a central government team of medical experts had started visiting Maharashtra on a fortnightly basis. They advised the state government that due to the rising number of Covid cases, the Centre believed that Mumbai could have as many as 1,00,000 cases by 31 May and would require 70,000 hospital beds. Perhaps 30,000 patients could be home-quarantined. The MCGM had only 3,000 beds in its hospitals. Newspapers had stopped being delivered. Television news channels showed daily images of makeshift tents that had been put up on open grounds for patients in Italy and Iran where the virus was raging, killing hundreds every day. The health infrastructure in Italy was at breaking point. Hospitals were refusing to admit all but critical patients.

The problem of availability of hospital beds, given Mumbai's population, was a big worry. The authorities did a rough calculation. Reveals Chahal: 'Till April, private hospitals were not on board. They came in only after 21 May. We had not thought that private hospitals would support us to the extent they did. Since Independence, not even once had private hospitals treated patients at government rates. But even then we realised that we'd be short of beds. As it happens, Chief Minister Uddhav Thackeray does a lot of research online. He advised us that we could build a Jumbo hospital on the BKC MMRDA grounds. The rest of us did not quite understand this idea. We could not imagine a functioning hospital on an open ground. But the CM had done his research. He said if they can set up functional field hospitals in China within weeks, why not in India?

'I had fair knowledge about this from my army background, having stayed in cantonment camps. I had seen huge field hospitals functioning in army tents. I knew that a hospital can function from an open ground if built with a solid foundation and structure. If the army can build hospitals and accommodation for troops on the border in such structures, then why can't we? Other MCGM officers could not fully reconcile to the idea of a hospital built on an open field. But I have actually seen army hospitals, offices and even residences functioning in such structures, built within days or weeks. When new regiments were raised near the border at Jodhpur and Bikaner, even the ammunition was stored in huge tent-like structures. When we had a meeting with the CM, I suggested we call in the army and request it to build the hospital structure. But that was not seen to be practical. The CM told me to instead contact the MMRDA, CIDCO and the municipal commissioners of Thane, Mira-Bhayander, Kalyan, etc. They should urgently give a list of all open grounds with them. Within days, every commissioner submitted his list of open plots. We found that the biggest open plot was at BKC. Nowhere in Mumbai was there a bigger plot than this.'

The MMRDA was called in and told that since it was the owner of the property, it should build the hospital there or outsource the contract. 'To build a field hospital you first needed a strong structure,' says Chahal. 'We had initially thought of a 1,000-bed hospital. We had to create an inventory of what was required. We finally built 2 hospitals—BKC 1 and BKC 2. Each has around 1,000 beds with a total of nearly 2,100 beds between them spread over 10 acres. The construction started around 25 April 2020. The inventory was created to take care of every requirement for the 2 hospitals to function efficiently. The idea was to build quarantine beds there. Nobody could imagine at that point in time that oxygen cylinders, ventilators or ICUs could function in a specially built field hospital.'

Contractors were appointed and told to lay a plinth. Engineers then erected a double-layered roof and walls made of strong canvas cloth material. 'When I took charge,' Chahal recalls, 'Covid-positive patients started increasing in huge numbers. Videos began appearing in social media about Mumbai's Covid plight. Hundreds of vulnerable slum dwellers were getting infected. The virus enters through your nose or mouth, lies in your throat and then, through the air pipe, enters your lungs and affects them, depending upon each person's immunity. There is no big hospital next to Dharavi. People from the slum virtually flooded Sion Hospital, the nearest medical facility. The dean of Sion Hospital was helpless. No beds were available. He would put an extra bed in the veranda or make 2 patients sleep on one bed. A video surfaced of that—2 people lying on one bed, and another of people lying on the floor. One day, a 100 patients came at the same time. There were no beds so they were told to lie on the floor and that they would be treated later. A video of this too went viral on social media.'

One day, several deaths of Covid-affected patients took place in Mumbai. The MCGM had only 80 operational ambulances at that time. They serviced as many as 120 hospitals. A dead body was taken out of the mortuary of one of these hospitals to be transported for the last rites. The staff waited for an ambulance to arrive. It took an hour to come. In the meantime, the hospital staff put the dead body in a body bag and placed it on a patient's bedside. A video of this again went viral, alleging that patients were made to lie next to a dead body. Social media exploded with such videos right through the summer of 2020.

'When these videos were getting posted, an idea struck me,' says Chahal. 'Construction of the new BKC 1 Jumbo hospital had reached a stage where the structure was ready. Beds had to be put in and furniture and medical equipment placed to make it functional. I proposed to the chief minister at a meeting that we should also build a Jumbo hospital at NESCO, Goregaon, another in Dahisar Naka, and yet others in Mulund Naka and Mahalaxmi Race Course.'

Chahal managed to convince the chief minister and the chief secretary that none of the proposed Jumbo hospitals should function as Covid Care Centres. They must, instead, be Dedicated Covid Health Centres (DCHCs) or Dedicated Covid Hospitals (DCHs). They must have oxygen beds and ICUs with ventilators, specialist doctors and dialysis facilities. The Jumbos could be custom-built for this category of patients as well.

Chahal urged the chief minister to not allow the city to waste its resources. Each Jumbo hospital was costing the BMC ₹150 crore to set up and run. The government was quick to accept the idea of building multiple Jumbo hospitals to treat Covid patients who were flooding private, government and municipal hospitals. It was decided that since the MCGM was fighting the Covid war on an emergency basis, no construction work should be given to the civic body itself. the CIDCO was entrusted with the construction of the Jumbo hospital at Mulund. The MMRDA had been asked to build the Jumbo hospital at BKC. Other Jumbo field hospitals at the Worli Dome, Byculla, the Mahalaxmi Race Course, NESCO Goregaon, Dahisar and elsewhere were outsourced to various established agencies.

Aaditya Uddhav Thackeray, minister for environment, tourism and protocol to the state government as well as guardian minister for Mumbai, pioneered the concept of the Worli Dome Jumbo field hospital purely through a CSR effort. This hospital, with more than 600 Covid beds, including Covid ICUs, was the first Jumbo field hospital to be established in Mumbai.

Says Chahal: 'This happened due to the untiring efforts of Aaditya Thackeray who has been hands-on, 24/7, in the fight against Covid right from day one. He possesses great qualities of head and heart and is an excellent team leader who carries everyone along in a seamless manner through his integrity and character. He is a role model for future young politicians of the country. Even though he got affected with Covid later, he never looked back and on recovery continued his visits to containment zones and slums in Mumbai almost on a daily basis. He possesses the qualities which would make him one of the tallest political figures in Maharashtra in the years to come. It is always a great pleasure working with him and taking things forward under his guidance. He exhibits the remarkably calm composure and maturity of a seasoned politician. His active, constant and unflinching support to me proved to be a game changer in Mumbai's fight against the Covid pandemic.'

Chahal wrote to all other municipal commissioners in the Mumbai Metropolitan Region (MMR) that 60 per cent of the beds in the Jumbo hospitals must be only oxygenated beds. This was acceptable to the government. The critical need for oxygen was recognised in Mumbai at an early stage, allowing it to tackle oxygen shortages a year later during the second wave that would prove far deadlier than the first wave and cause four times as many daily fatalities. For the moment though, all minds were focused on the ongoing first wave of the pandemic, which was now in its third virulent month.

Various agencies entrusted with building the Jumbos were told to create large oxygen tanks. Initially, the MCGM chipped in by creating oxygen tank facilities in the BKC, Worli Dome and NESCO Goregaon Jumbos. These would prove invaluable in the larger crisis that lurked, as yet unseen. 'If we needed oxygenated beds,' says Chahal, 'then there were two options: one, get a truckload of cylinders every day; and two, keep oxygen tanks there in silos. We knew we were going to fight the Covid battle for years. So we gave the work to build these oxygen tanks to contractors. We called a 48-hour tender. They are huge silos, as big as a multi-storey building. All these facilities were converted into oxygen tank facilities by the MCGM. Pipelines were laid next to each Jumbo hospital bed. Each bed was given an oxygen connection. It was a great engineering feat.

'Out of 1,000 beds in BKC 1, around 600 beds were fitted with oxygen pipes. All this took place within a few days. It was a war against Covid-19 and we had to be quick. After this, I proposed to the CM that we should plan ICUs as well in at least some of these Jumbo hospitals. We could then upgrade them to Dedicated Covid Hospitals (DCHs) where there are ventilator beds and ICU beds. In Worli Dome, Aaditya Thackeray, played a proactive role. He urged a few corporate houses to get involved and provide portable ICUs. These can hold up to 30-35 beds and are functioning even today in portable containers. The containers are imported. Each container has 2-4 beds. There are 612 ICUs functioning in Worli Dome, BKC 1, BKC 2, NESCO and Mulund. All these Jumbo field hospitals were built with ICU beds nearly a year before the second crippling wave struck Mumbai. We were ready. 4 more Jumbos were built in July-October 2021 during the second wave of the pandemic to take care of future emergencies. This increased the number of functioning Jumbo field hospitals in Mumbai to 11 with advanced facilities and paediatric beds. Today, Mumbai has 15,200 Covid beds and 1,402 ICU beds in 11 Jumbo hospitals.

'We established dialysis beds as well in the Jumbo field hospitals. By September 2020, we had 612 ICU beds functioning in the Jumbos.

We also converted quarantine beds into new ICU dialysis beds in Jumbos across the city. This has been a great experience for Mumbai as no other city built ICU dialysis beds in brand new field hospitals. We constructed the world's largest Jumbo field hospital in NESCO; Goregaon. It is spread over 20 acres. Large exhibitions used to be held there. We installed a total of 3,000 beds, including 1,800 oxygen beds and 224 ICU bed, there. It is the largest Covid hospital in the world with ICU beds functioning today as well. NESCO is even bigger than BKC 1 and BKC 2 which together have around 2,100 beds. All our Jumbos are centrally air-conditioned. We appointed several agencies for catering, housekeeping, laundry, air-conditioning, gas supply and so forth. Multiple outsourced agencies were deployed. These Jumbo field hospitals are like 5-star medical facilities, at par with many leading private hospitals.'

Shortage of hospital beds was endemic across India, especially in large cities. To ensure that Mumbai did not fall short of beds, the MCGM made provisions for additional beds across its own hospitals and the new Jumbos. 'The capacity of over 15,200 beds in our 11 Jumbos now exceeds what is available in Mumbai's 144 private hospitals put together,' says Chahal. 'Initially everybody was sceptical about the Jumbo field hospital idea. In June 2020, when NESCO Goregaon was about to become functional, a well-known former TV journalist who has an online video platform, called me saying, "Mr Chahal, you have created thousands of beds which will not be utilised. You have created white elephants." When beds were not available, journalists were criticising us. Now the same journalists, when beds were available, were calling them white elephants. I told her that this is a war we are fighting. I wish the beds would remain empty forever but not even one citizen of Mumbai should be denied a fully equipped hospital bed if he or she needs it.'

As the first wave of the pandemic spread, Chahal requested the chief minister to talk to the founder of Asian Heart Institute, Dr Ramakanta Panda. 'His hospital is just 50 metres across the road from the BKC Jumbo,' says Chahal. 'He has a 15-bed ICU. No patient, at the time of the pandemic's peak, was coming for non-Covid procedures. Dr Panda's ICU was lying shut. The senior doctors were sitting at home. So I proposed the idea of temporarily establishing our Covid ICUs there as well. We requested Dr Panda to give us his ICUs to use for a few weeks.

'Our construction of ICUs at the Jumbo hospitals carried on simultaneously. ICU construction is a major challenge—all ICU beds come from abroad. They are specialised beds. We don't manufacture them in India. These beds are fitted with inbuilt advanced medical equipment. We floated tenders for 2-3 days at a stretch for hundreds of ICU beds. It took us time to procure all this material and the procurement went on till September 2020. ICUs are highly complicated. There are advanced monitors, special suction machines and other sophisticated medical equipment. Dr Panda graciously agreed that we could add his existing ICUs to the BKC Jumbo inventory till our imported ICU beds arrived. Having an ICU medical facility next door to our Jumbo field hospital was a great psychological reassurance to Covid-19 patients. The chief minister called Dr Panda for a meeting. Dr Panda agreed to share his ICUs with us for as long as we wanted. We remain grateful to Dr Panda and his doctors. We continued using Dr Panda's ICUs from June to August 2020 during the most critical phase of the first wave. Thus, from 1 June, we could announce that the BKC 1 Jumbo field hospital had become a DCH-level hospital with fully functional ICUs for Covid-19 patients.'

For the commissioner, another challenge, however, lay ahead: the unpredictable Mumbai monsoon. Says Chahal: 'I have lived for the last 30 years in Mumbai and know what the monsoons are. I have seen that terrible day, 26 July 2005, when the whole of Mumbai was literally under water. I was worried about what would happen to our Jumbo field hospitals if there were floods during the monsoon. The location of the BKC Jumbo hospital is exactly 50 metres from the banks of the Mithi River. I told my team that we have patients lying on beds 50 metres from this river which is known for flooding every year. Our engineering department got to work. It fitted dewatering pumps all around the BKC Jumbo hospital. The Mithi River went above danger levels 3 times during the monsoon. But the pumps functioned well and did their job. The plinth was fairly high above the ground level. Before the water could enter the hospital, our pumps flushed it out.

'Dewatering pumps were planned in all our field hospitals. There was no flooding in NESCO, Worli Dome and Mahalaxmi. The main problem was at BKC, Dahisar Naka and Mulund Naka which are low-lying areas. But we had pumps everywhere. Not even a drop of water entered these Jumbos—not even in August 2020, which was the wettest month on record in the last 65 years, nor in September 2020, the wettest September in many, many years. Amidst all this we had a cyclone threat on 3 June. But in the end all was well.'

Recruiting doctors to man the Jumbo field hospitals was the next immediate task. By 1 June 2020, the field hospitals were ready. On 8 June, the 24 war rooms were in place with pre-MBBS students monitoring patient logistics from there. But the Jumbo hospitals needed senior qualified doctors to take care of the Covid patients admitted there. Chahal again turned to Dr Lahane and asked: where can we get so many specialists, MD doctors, MS doctors, MBBS doctors, to run these Jumbo field hospitals?

Chahal spent sleepless nights pondering over the availability of doctors and the need to expand the city's health infrastructure to meet the Covid challenge. The capacity of the 7 Jumbos at the time was 9,275 beds. A large number of highly qualified senior doctors, medical and paramedical personnel, health workers and nurses were needed to treat the influx of patients, many needing specialised care in ICU beds. The MCGM clearly needed to come up with innovative ideas. The number of Covid-positive cases was surging and there was a sense of growing panic in the city.

During the first lockdown, Chief Minister Uddhav Thackeray frequently communicated through live Facebook briefings. On seeing these briefings, Chahal had a eureka moment on solving the critical issue of recruiting additional senior doctors to man the newly set up Jumbo field hospitals. He recalls: 'There are large numbers of retired doctors from the army, navy, air force, central and state governments, medical colleges, government hospitals, private hospitals, etc. They are a resource. I requested the CM to address them on his next Facebook Live broadcast and tell them to please come forward. We will pay ₹80,000 per month to MBBS doctors, ₹2 lakh per month to specialist MD doctors and even more to super-specialist doctors.'

The CM duly announced on his next Facebook Live broadcast that retired senior doctors and other medical personnel who would like to help in the Covid-19 crises should come forward and register themselves on a specially designated email id which the MCGM had created. The response was extraordinary. More than 3,600 doctors, nurses and paramedics mailed their biodata. From the applicants, over 570 senior doctors, paramedics and nurses were deployed in the Jumbo field hospitals in a matter of weeks. They were given a list of Jumbo centres they could operate from, depending on which part of Mumbai they lived. Prajakta Lavangre, a young IAS officer, handled this work, Chahal notes, with extreme efficiency.

'In the second phase, we focused on recruiting and deploying additional nursing staff in the Jumbos,' says Chahal. 'All our medical colleges and hospitals—KEM, Nair, Sion, Cooper—have nursing institutes. Dr Lahane told me that there are a number of girls doing a nursing course. A final year batch was waiting for the last exam to be conducted.

There were 600 nursing students in that batch. We immediately took them on board. Fully qualified, bar sitting for their final exam, they were paid a monthly sum equivalent to what was paid to a certified nurse. Thus, 600 additional nurses came on board virtually overnight. All were deployed in the Jumbos. We now had a total of nearly 1,200 doctors, paramedics and nurses for our new field hospitals.'

Next, Chahal reached out to the Kerala governments seeking another 100 doctors and nurses who had actually done Covid-related work in the state that had been the first in India to be struck by the virus in January 2020. Chahal sought the medicos from Kerala on loan to Maharashtra. 'I wrote an emotional letter to the Kerala government and spoke to them on the phone,' he says. 'Dr Lahane, as director of medical education in Maharashtra, meanwhile, spoke to the director of medical education in Kerala. In my letter, I wrote that we would learn from their doctors. They would be of great help in the crisis. We said we will pay for their transportation, drive them in AC buses from Kerala to Mumbai and put them up in 5-star hotels. They would travel in AC buses from their hotels to the hospitals they were assigned to and back to their hotels every day. We got 100 doctors and nurses from Kerala through this initiative. Many were very senior doctors who were deployed in various hospitals on Covid-19 duty.'

As more Jumbo hospitals became operational, Chahal knew they would need an even greater number of medical personnel at various levels. He spoke to state minister for medical education, Amit Deshmukh. Says Chahal 'I requested him to give me doctors on loan from Wardha, Beed, Yeotmal and Latur where no cases existed at that time. I told him that I did not want specialised doctors. I needed residents who are doing a 3-year MD or MS course, post-MBBS. They are there 24 hours a day. They are on the verge of becoming MD, MS, surgeons, physicians. They are paid ₹55,000 per month. I requested the minister to give me 50 doctors from Beed, 50 from Latur, 50 from Wardha and 50 from Yeotmal since there were no Covid cases in these places in mid-2020. They also had no work at that point. If he loaned them to us, we could deploy them quickly in Mumbai where there was a dire need. The former minister went out of his way and gave me 150 doctors who were in their final year of MD and MS at medical colleges. Dr Lahane, who was in charge of medical postings, assigned them to Mumbai. They stayed at 5-star hotels. These 150 doctors also became a part of our healthcare system across both our Jumbos and traditional hospitals, and helped us to contain the first wave of the pandemic and prepare ourselves for a possible second wave.

'Thus, a total of over 1,500 newly recruited doctors and paramedics, along with more than 9,000 new Jumbo hospital beds, became a major asset in Mumbai's Covid-19 fight. All the 612 ICUs in Jumbo hospitals were outsourced to groups of medical professionals in September 2020 and this mechanism will continue till necessary to overcome the paucity of experts required to run ICUs. The entire medical manpower was created in a matter of a month during the first wave of this pandemic in the summer of 2020. It was akin to putting both the hardware and software in place. First, the hardware: construction of all 7 Jumbos and their complex engineering, oxygen pipelines and ICUs; and second, the software, recruiting qualified medical personnel to manage it all.'

Chahal often uses human psychology to achieve his objectives. 'A person,' he says, 'cares not just about salary. Status is equally important. So during one of our Zoom meetings, I remarked that Cooper Hospital has 500 beds, KEM has 800 beds, Sion has 700 beds. But each of our Jumbo hospitals has around 1,000 beds at least. I now wanted a dean for each. These Jumbo centres are bigger than our government and private hospitals. There should surely be a dean for these Jumbos too. All the deputy deans—or equivalents—at KEM, Sion, Nair, Cooper and 7 Hills should volunteer. They may have not become deans in their lifetime. Now was an unexpected opportunity. All the Jumbo hospitals were ready to be operationalised with medical personnel. But how do you run them without a dean? If patients start dying there because of poor facilities or management, then what do you do?

'Dr Lahane was not attached to the MCGM but he was more loyal to me than anyone else due to our old relationship. Human relationships are very important in a crisis. This played a major role in harnessing the huge medical staff of thousands of doctors and nurses in brand new hospitals set up in record time on open grounds. We, therefore, decided that any doctor heading our Jumbo hospitals in BKC, NESCO and elsewhere would be given the official designation—by order—of dean of the hospital. The dean shall enjoy all powers of procurement and of administration—whatever a dean of, for example, KEM has today. If a patient is admitted, the dean of KEM can buy medicine worth crores of rupees without informing me. I said that the deans of the new Jumbo hospitals will be equivalent to him.

'When this proposal was put forward, senior doctors in government hospitals voluntarily agreed to act as deans in the Jumbos. Their salaries would remain the same as in their previous posts but they would get enchanced status and tremendous powers of administration and procurement. The Jumbo deans would be the principal decision-makers in their field hospitals. Many of these new deans have subsequently, in the past more than a year, proved that they have both administrative skills and medical knowledge. This is how each of the Jumbos in Mumbai got a dean and became a full-fledged hospital.'

The new deans in fact, went one step ahead in managing the Jumbos. Given independent power, they began innovating. 'They are intelligent with a lot of experience,' Chahal points out. 'I was pleasantly surprised one day when I visited one of the Jumbos. It was running aerobic classes for asymptomic patients who did not require oxygen. Patients in other Jumbos were doing yoga and meditation. This had psychological benefits for patients. The new deans had created all this without my knowledge. They had the power to troubleshoot every problem on their own. The initiative of making them deans has proved to be a great success and made our Jumbo field hospitals function professionally.'

To boost the morale of MCGM workers, many of whom had died during the pandemic's first wave, Chahal issued a memo on 20 September 2020 to set the record straight as the pandemic began to wane: 'I wish to share that in the last 31 days, from 20 August to 20 September, 2020, the average Covid death rate under the MCGM has come down to 2.2 per cent and the overall Covid death rate under the MCGM has consequently fallen. We have started monitoring the weekly mortality rate every Monday morning, covering all public and private hospitals, and this has resulted in a drastic fall in the mortality rate. We are striving to bring the average mortality rate per day further down in the next 30 days.

'Besides this, due to our enhanced testing, even though the number of cases has increased from an average of 1,000 per day to approximately 2,000 per day, we still have 4,777 Covid beds and 271 ICU beds vacant as on yesterday, ensuring smooth patient management through our 24 ward war rooms. Our Jumbo field hospitals have now started working under the mentorship of eminent and expert doctors from private hospitals like Breach Candy, Bombay Hospital, Hinduja, Lilavati, Nanavati, Fortis, etc. since last week. I'm grateful to 35 top doctors from these hospitals who will guide our doctors at the Jumbo hospitals for patient treatment through telephonic medical guidance, and occasional visits, to reassure Jumbo hospital patients.'

The MCGM's series of innovations drew praise from unexpected quarters. Former IAS officer Anil Swarup explained[9] how Mumbai had emerged from a public health crisis:

[9]The *Daily Guardian*, 22 September 2020.

'Mumbai has been in the news for all the wrong reasons in the recent past. Even before that, it appeared that the relentless march and the devastating consequences of Covid-19 couldn't be taken care of in the metropolis. It spread like wildfire during the last week of April 2020. The slums of Mumbai, especially Dharavi, Govandi and Deonar, were impacted. On account of limited testing facilities and a short supply of COVID beds in the city of Mumbai, there were a number of deaths. Some dead bodies were even found on the streets and road dividers. One of the biggest slums of Asia, Dharavi, with a population of 8,00,000, was visibly out of control. There were only around 3,700 Covid beds available in the city and approximately 1,500 people were reporting positive every day.

'Social media was replete with videos depicting dead bodies on the road, more than one patient lying on a hospital bed, dead bodies kept on hospital beds next to alive patient on the bed, etc. Infected patients from the slums of Mumbai were flocking hospitals gasping for breath and were dying within a few hours of reaching a hospital. The death rate had gone beyond 8 per cent. The Municipal Corporation of Greater Mumbai (MCGM) had only 480 ICU beds, 80 ambulances and four hearse vehicles for deceased Covid-19 patients. When the Central Government Covid-19 Monitoring Team arrived at Mumbai on 5 May 2020, it pointed out glaring deficiencies in Mumbai and how things were getting out of control. It added that Mumbai would explode, leading to thousands of deaths in the near future.

'There was utter mismanagement and deficiency of resources in the fight against Covid-19 in Mumbai. Even the media started raising the demand of handing over Mumbai to the army to combat Covid-19. Mumbai had become the hotspot in the country. There was panic all around and a sizeable number of citizens of Mumbai were fleeing to safer places. Sheer helplessness provided ready fodder for the national media as well. All this resulted in tremendous pressure on the state government. Left with not many options, the state government shifted the incumbent municipal commissioner even before he had completed a year in this assignment. In his place an IAS officer, Iqbal Singh Chahal, was asked to take over.

'Greater emphasis was laid on testing. Arrangements were made to ensure that results of the tests were made available within 24 hours. Mumbai became the only city in the country where all tests report would come within this period without exception. More than 7.50 lakh RT-PCR tests, which is the gold standard, were conducted in the city. This is one of the highest in the country. With more than a ten-fold increase in the number of ambulances from 80 to 825, it was ensured that they were available on call. A huge pool of trained paramedics and doctors was created in the city. This was achieved by hiring retired doctors from the defence services as well as the State and Central Government. More than 100 doctors and nurses were sourced from Kerala on loan. Around 800 MBBS intern students were deployed to manage the ward war rooms. IAS officers were drafted to oversee daily administration of major hospitals in Mumbai. Consequent to these efforts, recoveries have gone beyond 80 per cent and the death rate that was initially 8 per cent in the month of April came down to almost half within a month and finally down to 1.8 per cent.'

The situation would improve further in the 5 months between 22 September 2020, when Swarup wrote this article, and 10 February 2021 by when cases and deaths in Mumbai had fallen to a nadir. Letting its guard down, Mumbai was whiplashed by an infectious and lethal variant that led to a debilitating second wave of the pandemic.

The second wave of Covid-19 struck Maharashtra without warning in February 2021. By 4 April, daily cases in Mumbai had climbed to over 11,000. Across Maharashtra, the situation was grim. Cases spiralled to nearly 70,000 in the state. Mumbai, Pune and Nagpur as well as rural areas were hit hard by the mutant variant, later dubbed Delta by the WHO. The health infrastructure built to combat the first wave would, however, stand the city in good stead.

'As far as medical infrastructure for the cascading waves of the pandemic is concerned,' notes Chahal, 'we built it and paid for it. Now recurring expenditure is basically on medicines and personnel. While subsequent third and fourth waves remain a concern, when the pandemic does finally ebb, the city's medical infrastructure, although created to fight Covid-19, will be a priceless post-Covid asset for all other diseases.

'Another advantage of the Covid Care Centres and the Jumbo field hospitals was that they became vaccination centres. They are hubs for vaccination across all morbidities, not just Covid. The Covid-19 vaccination programe will, in any case, go on in this country well into 2022. We have to vaccinate a large section of India's 1.35 billion people, including children below the age of 18. There's a long way to go. Bill Gates said that it would be end-2022 by the time the vaccination programme covers both urban and rural India for all adults and children. The Jumbos are multi-use facilities. Their utility value will be long-lasting—during public health emergencies and in the normal course of medical care as well. The Jumbo medical facilities are a case study for the country.

'Many patients say they prefer to be treated at the Jumbos rather than, for example, at KEM, Nair or Sion Hospitals. The Jumbo hospitals are centrally air-conditioned, impeccably clean, stock every medicine available in other hospitals, and outsource laundry and housekeeping to professional agencies. Facilities at the Jumbos are more thoroughly sanitised than those in many municipal and government hospitals.'

Chahal adds: 'Besides, patients had come to realise that ICUs in particular were very well managed in the Jumbos. This was a critical factor during and after the highly infectious second wave of the pandemic. Top doctors and specialists from private hospitals continue to visit those Jumbos that are operational. Through a mentoring programme, the Jumbos are attached to some of the most prestigious private hospitals in the city and they had become very sought after. The treatment and stay was totally free. Several Bollywood stars, private sector executives and even income-tax commissioners have been treated here. The Jumbos are well-equipped and brand new from inside. I organised a visit of doctors from Breach Candy and Bombay Hospitals to the BKC Jumbo. Later we took two high court judges to the BKC Jumbo. They all said that the Jumbo medical centre was like a 5-star hospital facility.'

The Jumbo field hospitals proved to be a game changer in Mumbai's fight against Covid-19. Their pathology lab testing and availability of drugs took the pressure off the city's traditional private and government medical facilities. By July-August 2020, with India still in the grip of the pandemic's first wave, the usage of antiviral drugs Remdesivir, Tocilizumab and Favipiravir had increased sharply. A Remdesivir injection was available at ₹16,000 for one vial. Tocilizumab cost ₹40,000 for one vial. Favipiravir was selling at ₹105 per tablet. The challenge for the MCGM was to make the procurement of these critical drugs affordable. Chahal told the additional municipal commissioner in charge of projects, P. Velarasu, who had helped procure ICU infrastructure for the Jumbos, to float tenders and quickly obtain quotations for drug procurement.

In May 2021, the WHO declared Remdesivir ineffective in the treatment of Covid-19. But the drug remained a popular mode of treatment for mild cases of Covid-19. Recalls Chahal: 'When Remdesivir emerged as the drug of choice for certain levels of Covid-19 infections, the US company Hetero had a monolpoly over the drug. That is why they were charging ₹16,000 per vial. We floated a tender and procured 3,000 vials of Remdesivir and started distributing them free of cost among government and MCGM hospitals as well as to the Jumbos. Similarly, we procured Tocilizumab at ₹40,000 per vial as well as Favipiravir and supplied them to all our hospitals, including the hospitals, for free. But we could not supply these medicines to private hospitals. There, patients were paying for these drugs at the higher rate and we could not fund them free of charge.

'The moment we procured the first lot of medicines, newspapers immediately reported that black marketing of the medicines had started. Complaints came to me that drugs costing ₹40,000 for one vial and given free of cost to KEM or Sion Hospital were being sold in the black market. Some private doctors in clinics could be charging ₹50,000 for one vial. Patients were ready to pay, this price as the virus had spread and vaccination was still a distant prospect. The WHO's declaration on the relative lack of efficacy of Remdesivir came later. Demand for the drug continued to soar. So did black marketing.'

In July 2021, KEM Hospital, which mostly treats critical patients, published a study that showed severely ill Covid-19 patients who were administered Remdesivir or Tocilizumab fared better than those who were not. As Yogita Rao reported[10]:

> 'The survival rate in patients receiving either or both the drugs was 64 per cent; it dropped to 34 per cent among those who did not get any of the two. In the group that benefitted, the rate of discharge among those given only Remdesivir was 66 per cent, for those who got only Tocilizumab it was 80

[10]The *Times of India,* 3 July 2021.

> per cent, and it was 47 per cent among those given both the drugs combined.
>
> 'The doctors studied the effect of Remdesivir and Tocilizumab on 521 patients at KEM Hospital and compared it with retrospective clinical details of 214 patients from a time when they were not available as experimental drugs for Covid (from 23 March to 31 May 2020). Of the 334 (64 per cent) patients discharged after being given either or both the drugs, only 5 needed supplemental oxygen. The doctors' observational study was published on 1 July 2021 in the *Journal of the Association of Physicians of India.*'

Black marketing of the three drugs, however, persisted. Innovation again took over. Chahal's team created a Google Drive linking the Jumbos with 26 hospitals. 'The dean uploaded the Google Drive every day with the number of Remdesivir and Tocilizumab vials with him,' says Chahal. 'A list was made of the patients who had already been given one vial each, along with their date of admission and date of discharge. Each dean had to daily record on his Google Drive the opening stock and the closing stock at 7.00 pm. I could monitor this in real-time on my computer. In this system, not a single vial would be leaked out in the black market. I wrote in my order that an audit will be conducted when the patients get discharged. Our teams would go to their homes and check whether they were given Remdesivir or not. Their relatives would be asked regarding the medication given to them. One cannot fudge figures. If the relatives said that no Remdesivir or Tocilizumab was given from beginning to end but the opposite was showing up in the Google Drive system, then a thorough investigation would take place. This system put an end to the black market for expensive imported drugs used to control the first wave of the pandemic. After the WHO advisory, however, the use of Remdesivir declined somewhat. But it remains in demand along with other Covid medicines. It continues to be used in mild-to-moderate cases of Covid-19.'

The demand for Remdesivir and Tocilizumab cut across the city's demographics. A senior Maharashtra state politican phoned Chahal late one evening and said his daughter-in-law was serious. He required a vial of Tocilizumab. He had called up all the hospital deans. No one was prepared to give him even one vial. They said if they did, they will be caught in the MCGM's online system. It would be difficult to justify where one vial had disappeared. Chahal told the senior politician not to blame the deans. Even he would not break protocol by phoning a dean and asking him to give a vial. Instead, Chahal said he would ring up Nikhil Chopra, then Cipla's CEO in India, and tell him to provide a vial directly from the company. Payment should be made directly to Cipla. The vial was arranged swiftly but without breaking protocol.

'The Google Drive worked well,' smiles Chahal. 'I can put on record that after the news story appeared on black marketing of Remdesivir and we created the Google Drive system the same evening, there has not been a second news item about black marketing of this medicine.'

By August 2020, when the first wave had peaked, all MCGM hospitals and Jumbos were well equipped with the three medicines. 'At one task force meeting which the chief minister attended,' Chahal recalls, 'Dr Shashank Joshi, a very eminent doctor, said that in his career of 40 years he had never seen municipal hospitals stocking critical medicines that private hospitals did not have.'

Admist all this, Chahal was struck by another idea. 'There are hundreds of hospitals in Mumbai—35 major, 75 smaller ones, hospitals in Thane and MMR—all were clamouring for these important pre-vaccine medicines,' he says. 'Before we got the vaccine, Covid patients perforce had to rely on these antiviral medicines. I requested Dr

Lahane to float a tender for these three critical drugs. He should quote huge volumes. Now that competition had come in—Cipla along with Hetero—we should go for volumes to reduce the price. He should open the best bid and flash the winning bid's cell number to the entire state of Maharashtra. Whoever wants the drugs can buy at this low price—whether it is a Thane hospital or a small hospital in Latur or Osmanabad. The CM approved the idea and instructed Dr Lahane to go ahead immediately. He floated tenders—Remdesivir for 25,000 patients, Tocilizumab for another 25,000 patients, and Favipiravir for yet another 25,000 patients. And the prices collapsed!

'We had procured Remdesivir for ₹16,000 per vial. It came down to ₹11,000 and then ₹4,000. It kept falling. Tocilizumab dropped from ₹41,000 per dose to ₹31,000. Favipiravir came down from ₹98 to ₹58. By doing this, 25,000 patients became relatively secure. The vendor's (the pharma company's name and mobile number were sent to all civil surgeons/collectors/municipal commissioners in Maharashtra as well as to private hospitals in Mumbai. There are about 150 hospitals in the city and scores of them in the rest of Maharashtra. Whoever wanted Remdesivir could ring up this number and pay directly at that rate. The process became streamlined and transparent. We flooded Maharashtra with these medicines. The idea worked and black marketing absolutely disappeared. The drugs started flowing into the market at affordable prices before vaccines became available in January 2021.'

Cipla had received a licence from the Indian government and the Drug Controller General of India (DCGI) to manufacture Remdesivir and Tocilizumab in India in Silvasa. 'That is also why the price of Remdesivir came down to ₹4,000 per vial at a crucial stage in October 2020 when we were just getting on top of the virus and a vaccine was still months away,' says Chahal

But the story could have taken a different turn. Chahal casts his mind back: 'It was around 7.00 pm on a Friday evening,

26 June 2020. Cipla's CEO Nikhil Chopra phoned me. He said he had imported intermediates from China to manufacture Remdesivir. The intermediates had landed at Mumbai's international airport's air cargo division. Now, this consignment could be used to manufacture one lakh Remdesivir vials for the entire country. But the Indian government had, meanwhile, banned 59 Chinese apps following the border clash in the Galwan Valley in eastern Ladakh on 15 June. Within weeks, orders were issued to ban key Chinese products in the country. The Union government further ordered that containers with Chinese products lying at Indian ports should meanwhile not be offloaded. Air cargos from China too, should not be released but sent back.

'When Nikhil Chopra called me, he said his intermediates to manufacture one lakh doses of Remdesivir had arrived from China but the principal commissioner of customs had refused to release the consignment. He said customs had received orders from the government. Chopra told me Cipla's licence would be of no use as only two countries in the world have the pharma intermediates needed for this drug—China and the US. Washington had put a ban on the export of this intermediate. If China's intermediates go back from Indian customs, Chopra said there will be zero local output of the drug.'

Chahal was worried. He knew he had to act quickly. 'I picked up the phone and called Union Finance Secretary Ajay Bhushan Pandey,' he recounts. 'We had worked together earlier. He was my senior by 5 years. I explained the entire issue and told him that I had spoken to the principal customs commissioner. The commissioner said verbal orders had come from the Central Board of Excise and Customs (CBEC), the controlling authority of customs. The chairman of CBEC had placed a block on the release of this China-origin consignment. The chairman of CBEC reports to Pandey. I requested Pandey to put in a word—thousands of lives would be saved. I sent Pandey a message at 5.47 pm on 26 June asking if I could call him. I again explained the situation to him. I told him that if the consignment of intermediates is not released, then we will not be able to manufacture this drug for at least the next 6 months. Nowhere else was this medicine available. In the absence of a vaccine, it was a key drug for Covid patients. Some very serious cases have been cured with this medicine. A vaccine was not yet in sight. Clinical trials were still on.

'Pandey is a chemical engineer from IIT. He told me to mail the name of the chemical formula of the ingredients. I immediately gave Pandey all the details, requesting him to again put in a word with the CBEC chairman. This message was sent on 26 June at 7.55 pm. Pandey did not call back. So the next morning, I called him. 27 June was a Saturday. Pandey told me that he had discussed my request with his team. But since there were a lot of problems with China, if we release the consignment and there is an issue with the intermediates, it will create havoc. Pandey was sorry but he could not release the intermediates. This interaction took place at around 11.30 am on 27 June.

'In the evening, we had a meeting at the mayor's old bungalow with the chief minister. Guardian Minister Aaditya Thackery, the then chief secretary Ajoy Mehta and a few others were present. I requested Mehta, Pandey's IAS batchmate, to speak to him. Mehta said he had spoken to Pandey. But the Union finance secretary was sceptical. Pandey said that China, following the Galwan Valley clash on 15 June, have could played mischief with the intermediates and it could even be virus-infected. He was not willing to release the consignment. I went to my office later on Saturday and called Cipla CEO Nikhil Chopra. I told him that the finance secretary of India is concerned about China potentially creating some problem with the intermediates. You are a world-class company, I said. Don't you have a high-tech lab in which you can identify a possible virus in the intermediates before you process it? Chopra said Cipla has one of the best labs in the world. It could identify any virus or contamination in the consignment. I requested Chopra to send me an email certifying this.

'The mail arrived at 9.15 pm on Saturday, 27 June. It stated that Cipla had the capability to identify any contamination or virus in these intermediates. There will be no problem if the intermediates are handed over to Cipla. It was like a guarantee. Now, in the Prime Minister's Office (PMO) there was a young IAS officer Shrikar Pardeshi. I had met him when he was a collector in Nanded. Elections were on and I had gone there as an observer on behalf of the Election Commission of India. Later, we worked together in Delhi. I sent an urgent email in his name as joint secretary to the Prime Minister's Office. I explained the entire situation in the mail. I also said that if the intermediate is released, it will not only benefit Mumbai but the whole of India. I enclosed Cipla's mail validating its confidence in identifying any potential contamination in the intermediates.

'Across India, lakhs of patients were using Remdesivir. So roughly one lakh doses in those critical times, June-July 2020, the first peak of the pandemic, could save thousands of lives. I literally begged the PMO to make an exception for these intermediates. After the young PMO officer received my mail, I spoke to him on the phone at around 10.00 pm. I requested him that whenever the prime minister is available, please tell him to read this mail. It is the urgent request of the commissioner, MCGM. Please just read this. After that, whatever his decision may be, it will be accepted, but first please read this mail. The PM should be aware of this dire situation.

'It was past midnight, I learnt later, when the young PMO officer showed my mail to the PM. The PM is very diligent. He works late every night. He read the mail just before 1.00 am. It was Saturday night. I was already asleep by 12.30 am. Next morning, at 9, I received a call from Vinayak Azad, the principal commissioner of customs, air cargo. He told me that instructions have been issued and we have released the intermediate consignment half an hour back as a special case. This was Sunday morning, 28 June, almost exactly 2 weeks after we lost 20 soldiers in the Galwan Valley clash with the People's

Liberation Army (PLA). To confirm this overnight development, I called Nikhil Chopra. He said, yes, Cipla's officer was on his way to the airport cargo section and the consignment will be with the company in another 30 minutes. All I can add here is: hats off to the PM. I salute him for taking it upon himself, at a time of a war-like situation with China, to take a decision at 1.00 am that could save, and did save, thousands of lives. Not many knew about this till now. The PM deserves the country's salutation.'

One item on the incident though did appear in the public domain at the time. India Today TV reported: 'Mumbai customs releases API for key Coronavirus drug after (MCGM) Chief's letter to the PMO.'

Meanwhile, there was a twist in the tale. The MCGM had floated tenders for 1,600 ICUs for its Jumbo field hospitals. Contractors who bid for the tenders and received contracts had ordered the ICU beds and ventilators from China. The high-tech Chinese beds had advanced inbuilt medical equipment. 'They too, were stuck at customs in the same manner as the drug intermediates,' says Chahal. 'So when the PM's message arrived that as far as Covid-19 is concerned, please release the intermediates' consignment, our Chinese-made ICU beds and ventilators also got released by customs. It would have been impossible to make these ICUs functional in our Jumbo field hospitals without all this equipment. It was a unique experience: we got life-saving drugs, saved human lives and we made our new Jumbo ICUs operational.'

As the third wave abated, nine of the eleven operational Jumbos were closed down. They had served the city well.

FOUR

THE MUMBAI MODEL

Though the first wave of the pandemic subsided by January 2021, the MCGM wisely decided not to close a single bed in its 7 Jumbo field hospitals in Mumbai. On 15 January 2021, the Jumbo at NESCO Goregaon had only 3 patients against a capacity of 3,000 beds with 224 ICU beds. The first wave resulted in 3,13,000 cumulative Covid cases in Mumbai out of which 11,400 passed away, establishing a mortality rate of 3.6 per cent. However, the second wave, despite its lethal virulence, resulted in a mortality rate of just 0.8 per cent in Mumbai, among the lowest for a global city of comparable size.

During the strong second wave of Covid-19, cases quadrupled in a matter of weeks. Deaths remained lower than in the first wave a year ago, but that was cold comfort. The highly infectious Alpha and Delta mutants ravaged the state. The lethality and infectivity of the B.1.617 variant that spread through Mumbai in February 2021, setting off a devastating second wave, can be gauged by comparing two sets of figures. On 3 July 2020, at the peak of the first wave, Mumbai had just 9,500 patients on hospital beds with 127 ICU beds vacant. On 30 April 2021, around the peak of the second wave, over 17,000 hospital beds were occupied by patients. Only 40 ICU beds were available despite the increase in beds across hospital categories.

Dr Soumya Swaminathan, chief scientist of WHO and former

director general of ICMR, wrote an important article in *India Today* in January 2021, weeks before the second wave struck India. She lauded India's fight against the coronavirus but urged caution as the battle would be a long and hard one. 'Covid-19 has been without a doubt the worst health crisis I have seen in my lifetime,' she conceded.

> 'I can't think of any other comparable event that has had this kind of debilitating impact on people, not just across one country but around the world. The first lesson of the pandemic was the lack of preparedness of health systems in countries across the world, including the most high-income ones. The gap was mainly in the area of public health—detection, surveillance, prevention and response to infectious disease threats.
>
> 'Systems need to be in place, including trained manpower, real-time data collection and analysis, quality-assured laboratories, a risk communication strategy and empowered health authorities who could advise the administration on action needed. Paradoxically, we have observed that some low- and middle-income countries, which relied less on high-tech and more on existing primary health and community-based approaches (like Rwanda, Senegal, Thailand and Vietnam), did relatively well.
>
> 'In India, there have been many positive developments. From just one laboratory, the National Institute of Virology, that could do the RT-PCR test in the beginning, today there are over 1,500 labs, both private and public, set up rapidly. This is also true of Personal Protective Equipment (PPE), which had to be imported initially but was soon being made indigenously. Also impressive was the innovation in diagnostic devices, analytical software and the use of artificial intelligence for exercises like contact tracing and detection of cases. Plus, several Indian companies are manufacturing vaccines, not

only by tying up with foreign groups but also by pursuing their own novel ideas. This has not happened before. All these show that there is a lot of potential and capacity, lessons that can be applied to other big public health problems.'

Meanwhile, with the Jumbo field hospitals up and running, Chahal turned his attention back to one of the most critical healthcare problems in Mumbai: its densely populated areas. Creating containment zones in chawls, shanties and slums was to be a priority throughout the pandemic. The coronavirus spreads from human to human. The WHO had prescribed a minimum physical distance of 1 metre between 2 people. In the tenements of Mumbai, where the density of population is very high, it was virtually impossible to maintain physical distancing. The prospect of the virus spreading was especially dire. Lessons had been learnt during the first wave but several problems remained intractable.

Due to low income levels, people living in small tenements found it difficult to buy santitisers, masks, protective equipment, gloves and medicines. 'These were major challenges for Mumbai,' says Chahal. 'International print and electronic media had reported that once the coronavirus enters India, the country would face a public health emergency.'

Turning thoughtful, Chahal reflects briefly on when he first realised the lethal potential of the coronavirus: 'My father-in-law, Ajit Singh Chatha, is an IAS officer. He retired as chief secretary of Punjab. Towards the end of December 2019, he warned me about the devastation that a new strain of an as yet undiscovered coronavirus could potentially cause in India. At that time, I was not aware of its full implications. It would soon be announced in China that Wuhan was going into a total lockdown because of a new highly infectious virus. My father-in-law then said that if this virus comes to India, it will be very difficult to stop it. It will create havoc in our country, especially in crowded cities. I did not react at the time but when the pandemic set in here, I remembered his words.'

Through the long pandemic, Chahal constantly worried about the challenge of imposing a lockdown in tenements and shanties where hundreds share a common toilet. 'You can enforce lockdowns in flats and bungalows where people have individual rooms,' he says animatedly. 'But not when 20 people share one room and sleep in shifts. I had visited the distant township of Malegaon where 28 people were staying in a single room. They were all bachelors with their families in Uttar Pradesh. They worked in the handloom industry in Malegaon. The room was rented. They would sleep in shifts; 7-8 people were always sleeping at a time. How do you impose a lockdown in such a situation?'

By mid-April 2020, the need for containment zones in Mumbai had become imperative. It would form an integral component of the Mumbai Model to control the pandemic through waves and surges in 2020 and 2021. The strategy was clear-eyed: if you cannot contain a small home with infected patients, you should contain an area to block the spread of the virus. It was decided to mark out areas with a population of 4,000-5,000. These could be rectangular or square and localised. The containment zone could thus cover around 1,000 families (assuming 5 people per family). The containment zone policy was drafted and constituted through various government guidelines. There was single-point entry and exit, and a plethora of other do's and don'ts for creating a containment zone.

'When I took over as commissioner on 8 May, the number of containment zones had reached 2,500,' recalls Chahal. 'There was no concept of a sealed building at the time. Even a building counted as a containment zone. This was creating a lot of confusion. So we brought in the concept of sealed buildings. With this, the number of containment zones fell to 1,000 in June 2020 during the peak of the first wave. Another 1,500 comprised sealed buildings. The 1,000 containment zones continued to present a huge challenge. In Dharavi, for example, there were dozens of containment zones.

'The biggest challenge was to manage the containment zones, do surveillance, and control the spread of the virus within the containment zones. Once the virus entered, it spread like wildfire. I visited a number of containment zones, beginning with Mukund Nagar in Dharavi. My next visit was to other containment zones like Govandi in Chembur, Deonar in M-East ward, again in the Chembur area, Juhu Jetty slums, then other Juhu slums, Worli slums, the Geeta Nagar slum in Colaba and the Appa Pada slum in Malad. We then went to slums in Goregaon and Borivili, the Kranti Nagar slums on the banks of the Mithi River and slums in Kalwa and Kalina. I visited 55 containment zones. In the slums, I would wear both a mask and a face shield. I was advised to wear double gloves and a surgical cap so as to not expose my skin to the virus.

'When I went to these containment zones, I could gather first-hand information on what was happening there. From April 2005 to August 2007, when the Maharashtra government decided to redevelop Dharavi, I was appointed as the officer on special duty (OSD) in charge of the Dharavi redevelopment project. I had used the opportunity to visit these areas in normal pre-pandemic times, and had a fair knowledge of the slums.'

When Chahal visited the slums for the first time as municipal commissioner, the knowledge he had absorbed over a decade ago as OSD for Dharavi's redevelopment enabled him to hit the ground running. 'I held meetings with my core team of additional commissioners, joint commissioners, zonal deputy commissioners and zonal ward officers,' he says. 'We selected and appointed a community leader in each of the 1,000 containment zones. The community leader could not be a politician or a local leader. He had to be a local living in that containment zone for many years, along with his family and children. That was a precondition I had laid down for selecting a community leader.

'We told our assistant commissioners—ward officers in charge of the 24 war zones—that this was a strict precondition. They already had a list of the 1,000-odd containment zones across the city which were under the MCGM at that time. I had separated the sealed buildings. We did not want to confuse sealed buildings with containment zones. They were to be addressed separately. This new concept of sealed buildings was not in the guidelines of the central government. By mid-May, Mumbai had demarcated containment zones and appointed community leaders—one for each containment zone. We decided that all community leaders should be given one free mobile phone on our behalf. Each of them was given the municipal commissioner's direct mobile number, the ward officers' mobile numbers and the ward war room's landline phone number.'

Dharavi and other slums in Mumbai have one unusual asset: around 1,500 doctors routinely practise in there thriving mini-cities in small 200 square feet clinics. They have MBBS or BMS degrees with one compounder each to assist them. The MCGM gave one week's advance quota of free PPE kits to each clinic. The protection encouraged these doctors to reopen their clinics which they had shuttered in panic when the pandemic first struck and a national lockdown was imposed. PPE kits worth several crore rupees were gifted to 1,500 local doctors in Dharavi and other slums in Mumbai. That in itself prevented the spread of serious infection among healthcare workers and saved countless lives.

Chahal adds: 'I told the community leaders that they have to report to the war rooms and the control room on whether these local doctors were opening their clinics or not. We did not want them to sit at home and sell the PPE kits, which they had received free from the MCGM, in the black market. In those days, PPE kits were very expensive and there was a thriving black market. So there was pressure on doctors, healthcare workers and sanitisation workers: if they cheated at their work, they would be caught. Despite the best efforts of Covid healthcare workers, if by chance a Covid patient was not given medical treatment, the community leader had to inform the relevant ward officers. They would immediately pick him up and take him to a hospital or a Covid Care Centre. These rules were given to community leaders and implementing them again proved tobe a game-changer.'

This was a classical case of management by decentralisation and delegation. Chahal elaborates: 'We told the community leaders that if the ward war rooms don't call you or if you call and they don't respond, then the next call should go directly to the municipal commissioner. Dharavi by now had dozens of containment zones. The community leaders started responding to us. Even the ward officers were apprehensive that if they did not respond to the community leaders, then the commissioner will come down heavily on them. So the whole system started working smoothly when the first wave of the pandemic was at its peak in June 2020 with nearly 1,00,000 daily positive cases nationwide and over 1,800 daily deaths.'

With the local doctors' clinics opening up and healthcare workers active in Mumbai's most congested areas, citizens became more aware of how to deal with the Covid-19 virus. Testing was simultaneously increased. It was clear that Mumbai's most vulnerable locations would need special attention through 2021 and well into 2022 till the pandemic lingered and vaccinations passed a critical level of 85-90 per cent of adults and children.

'A large number of teachers were deployed in the containment zones,' says Chahal, emphasising the long-term nature of the task that confronted the city as it fought to control the virus. 'Once the community leaders were selected, we gave them several orders in writing. First, the community leaders will interact with teachers in the local wards. Mobile numbers of the community leaders and teachers were exchanged. The responsibility for each containment zone was distributed among the teachers. Ward officers did a great job and syncronised this process. The system started functioning well. By 15 June the protocol had become very robust.'

Questions raised by critics centred around whether community leaders were themselves active and functioning. 'The question of not functioning does not arise,' Chahal responds, 'since every community leader is called several times in a day by our monitoring teachers even today. They simply cannot afford to be non-functional. Ward officials also have to visit slums and check on the work of community leaders. Of the MCGM's more than 1,08,000 employees, 500 work in the head office. All the others are in the field. So the MCGM has a hidden army of over one lakh workers. A ward officer has 4,000-plus employees under him. So the teams visiting the tenements and slums and checking on everything—whether authentic information is coming in or not—have substantial manpower. Besides this, we have deployed and joined hands with a large number of NGOs. They also give us feedback. For example, Bharatiya Jan Sangathna adopted auto rickshaws. If they find a positive case anywhere, they call the adopted autorickshaw for a pick-up and drop the patient into a nearby Covid Care Centre. The patient does not need an ambulance! He reaches a medical facility within a very short period of time.

'We told the NGOs that we do not have doctors to spare. So they built their own team of doctors. Many of these doctors were not living in or near tenements or slums, but they gave their services to patients in those areas free of charge. Philanthropists also started coming forward. The Rotary and Lions Clubs joined hands and gave us doctors who were willing to work in slums. More than 150 doctors worked in Dharavi during the peak of the pandemic in the first and second waves.'

The civic body's containment zone and war room strategies

attracted the attention of Harvard University. Says Chahal: 'I received a call from Harvard. They want to come to Mumbai and do a case study here for 7-10 days on the Mumbai Model. The containment zones were a critical component in the Mumbai Model to successfully control the second wave. If we had allowed the virus to grow during the second wave in mid-2021, it would have become like a volcano and burst. The second wave presented a major health challenge, but by then we had our medical infrastructure and manpower in place. As it turned out, the 24 war rooms and thousands of containment zones across the city, in slums, high-rises and elsewhere, were crucial in mitigating the virus' surge in the second and subsequent waves.'

Chahal constantly returns to the theme of Mumbai's slums in general, and of Dharavi in particular, for good reason. When the pandemic struck, he knew instantly that to control the spread of Covid-19 in the sprawling metropolis, controlling it in its slums, shanties, chawls and tenements was critical. The success of the Mumbai Model depended to a large extent on the success of the Dharavi Model.

Chahal made it a point to walk through the containment zones in all the slum areas during the peak of the pandemic. 'I would park my car outside them and walk inside,' he says. 'Your visibility is very important. People see that the municipal commissioner is checking on things personally, and they feel reassured. It also won the hearts of the slum dwellers. They started responding to our requests to cooperate on treatment, both in our new Jumbo field hospitals and in municipal, government and private hospitals. This was not just a medical issue. These were human beings watching terrible things happening around them to neighbours and friends who tested positive and died. When I went to the containment zones, I made it a point to visit a slum dweller's home. I would enter the public toilet, enter the doctor's clinic, enter a paan shop, a *kirana* store, a restaurant, a small workshop and ask them what problems they were facing.

'Gradually, these slum dwellers became reassured. They started cooperating with our officials who visited them to check on their health. A cordial relationship developed between the residents and the corporation's healthcare workers. There was not a single incident of violence against our officials. The slums have criminal gangs of every kind. Violence is never far from the surface. But today, my officers and I can go to any slum without security, and we will not be harmed.'

In the last week of June 2020, Chahal recalls, as the first wave continued unabated, 'We entered a containment zone in Appa Pada slum in Malad which was badly affected. It had more than 100 positive cases in a population of around 4,000 people. We went through the lanes and bylanes. As we moved further inside, the crowd became thinner and thinner. We were 5-6 officials at that point. I went into a very narrow lane. My officers told me not to go there as there could be security issues. It was a notorious slum. I told everyone to stay back. Only one ward officer, one police personnel and I went further in. It was a 3-foot-wide lane with an overflowing gutter. If you go forward 100-150 metres, you come up against a dead end. Then you have to find another narrow bylane to reach the required area.

'After walking for 8-10 minutes, I decided to inspect a public toilet along the way to see if it was being sanitised six times a day as per our protocol. Some residents nearby confirmed it was. We then entered a slum dwelling. It was just one room with a person lying on a bed. He did not have a door, only a curtain which was like a door for him. When we entered, he got up and sat on the bed. I asked him his name. He said it was Tiwari. We asked him if the toilet next door was being sanitised six times a day. He said yes. We asked him about the quality of food packets being delivered. He said the food packets were good and he was receiving them regularly. Then I asked him some more questions. I was wearing a mask, gloves, a surgical cap and a face shield. He said he was being well-looked-after. The first wave of the pandemic was still raging. But our surveillance mechanism had become so robust that it was now the backbone of our strategy to eradicate the virus from the slums. The interaction with Tiwari gave us hope that we were on the right path. Suddenly, the ward officer told Tiwari that it's the municipal commissioner who's talking to you. Tiwari promptly asked me if I was Chahal Sahab. I was surprised that he knew my name.'

The containment zone protocol applied to every citizen. For example, both the bungalows of the Bachchan family were declared "containment zones" and sealed during the first wave of the pandemic. In the second wave, hundreds of high-rise buildings were sealed as more cases emerged from affluent households than from slums or chawls.

Dharavi continued to be a signature success story right through Mumbai's long battle against the virus. 9 months after the pandemic first struck Mumbai, IANS reported on 25 December 2020: 'In what could be termed a "Christmas present" for the MCGM, Asia's largest slum, Dharavi, recorded zero cases on Friday—the first time since the first Covid-19 case and fatality appeared in Dharavi on 1 April. At one point, Dharavi ranked as the worst hotspot and the most worrisome for health authorities, but Dharavi now has a mere 12 active cases currently under treatment in local hospitals. "We salute the people of Dharavi for their full cooperation, following the MCGM's SOPs and other health guidelines that has helped immensely," an elated Municipal Commissioner I.S. Chahal told IANS. "This is a major achievement since the first case and death was reported from Dharavi on 1 April. All our efforts to control the pandemic here have yielded fruitful results."'

Dharavi also continued to attract global attention even as variants of the coranavirus led to a spike in cases worldwide. The Philippines announced that it would implement a similar model to control the contagion in the less affluent districts of Manila. At that time, a pleased

Chief Minister Uddhav Thackeray observed that 'Dharavi has now emerged as a global role model in tackling the coronavirus pandemic.'

Dharavi could have been a time bomb. The way it was defused is one of the defining stories of the years-long battle against the Covid pandemic. After receiving early praise, international recognition of Dharavi's continuing battle against Covid-19 gathered momentum. Nearly 6 months after the pandemic first struck Dharavi, the Australian Broadcasting Corporation (ABC) remarked[11]:

> 'As the coronavirus ran rampant, the largest slum in Asia decided to save itself. Many thought that it would be devastated,but after some initial problems, the model used there to prevent the spread of the virus has been such a success that the world needs to copy it.'
>
> The ABC report noted: 'With narrow streets, congested housing, underfunded healthcare and poor sanitisation, many thought that India's largest slum would be devastated by Covid-19. In fact, Dharavi, located in the financial capital Mumbai, is often heralded as a prime example of why the country was ill-prepared to deal with the coronavirus.'

The stigma associated with the disease affected morale the most in vulnerable neighbourhoods. 'Everyone was scared and locked themselves up in their homes,' remembers Chahal. 'Local residents told the ABC that when the coronavirus was spreading in our local areas, we felt Dharavi was going to be finished. At the time, Dharavi had recorded a few cases but the heathcare system was already struggling to keep up. Patients would be refused admission to hospitals and ambulances went missing in action. Residents complained that quarantine facilities lacked basic necessities and cleanliness. One person interviewed by the BBC, said:

[11]9 August 2020.

> '"I could not stand properly, I was vomiting and shivering, I lay down on the ground in the hospital, so many patients were coming in the hospital but did not get admission as beds were not available. Soon after me, my wife and child tested positive and were taken to various quarantine shelters. Corona was not just killing me, but killing my family. I lost hope for my survival and left it to God." Then he told the reporter that the authorities got on the front foot by knocking on doors and testing. Much has changed in Dharavi since the early outbreak. The entire neighbourhood seems to be winning the battle against the virus and its mutant variants.'

The Mumbai Model was soon the toast of the world. The *New York Times, the Wall Street Journal* and *The Economist* wrote copiously on the city's unique containment strategy and its long-term success as the pandemic waxed and waned. Crew from the BBC and the CNN filmed the developing story as the world fought the worst public health crises in a century. The World Bank once again joined the growing global media chorus. On 7 October 2020 it publicly recognised Mumbai's relentless battle against Covid-19 in tenements across the city. It said the success stemmed from a combination of customised solutions, community involvement and perseverance.

The World Bank pointed out that nearly a million people live in small tenements and dilapidated buildings with narrow lanes, bylanes and open sewers. To tackle Covid successfully in such a challenging environment is a testament to the city's chase the virus policy. In its Poverty and Shared Prosperity report, the World Bank reiterated that by tapping into the skills and dedication of community members, Mumbai city officials were able to stem the rapid spread of Covid-19 in vulnerable areas. NGOs and volunteers provided thousands of household items along with ration kits.

After reporting zero cases on Christmas Day, 25 December 2020, Dharavi reported zero deaths for another 75 days. But unbeknownst to the relieved city, where overall deaths had fallen to single digits in January and early February 2021, a deadly new mutant strain of the coronavirus lay in wait. It would wreak havoc in the second wave of the pandemic.

Chahal asks rhetorically: 'What was the difference in the MCGM's approach during the first wave in 2020 and the second wave in 2021? First, chase the virus with tracking, testing and treating; second, develop strategic public private partnerships. These remained common themes in both waves. We decided to do proactive screening in high-risk zones and organise fever clinics and camps to identify cases and manage key treatments. We mobilised all available medical practitioners. Many doctors came forward and the MCGM provided them with thermal scanners, pulse oximeters, masks and gloves. We started testing in high-risk zones. All the risks were carefully identified. Team MCGM has been outstanding throughout. Ashwini Bhide, P. Velrasu and Suresh Kakani, all additional municipal commissioners, performed remarkably well. They became my eyes and ears. I owe my success to their stellar performance.

'All medical practitioners were asked to communicate to the MCGM every possible Covid case. We sanitised the private clinics of all the local doctors. As we set up the health infrastructure in the slums, all the private hospitals came on board and were ready to treat patients. Sai Hospital in Dharavi, Prabhat Nursing Home and one other family nursing hospital were taken over by the MCGM and run by us. Since home quarantine was never an option in tenements and slum areas, the focus was on setting up maximum institutionalised quarantine facilities, covering all available schools, marriage halls, sports complexes, etc.'

In these institutional quarantine facilities, specific facilities were provided:

1. A community kitchen for breakfast, lunch and dinner;
2. 24/7 doctors, nurses, and medical staff;
3. Medicines;
4. All medical equipment.

A 200-bed Covid Care Centre hospital was set up with oxygenated beds within 14 days in Mahim Nature Park, Dharavi. This was even before the BKC Jumbo field hospital was built. The first Covid case was treated in that new Covid Care Centre weeks before the BKC Jumbo centre became functional. There was a strict enforcement of containment laws were implemented. Only critical patients were moved outside the slums for treatment. Over 90 per cent of the patients were treated inside slum areas.

Chahal elaborates on the strategy: 'The high-risk zones were sealed from all sides with the community leaders of the containment zones acting as Covid Warriors. We distributed 21,000 food packets (lunch and dinner) and 21,000 grocery and ration kits every single day free of cost to the residents of Dharavi. This ensured that people stayed inside their homes, reducing the risk of infecting others if they were asymptomatic carriers.'

Long before the second wave struck, however, Dharavi experienced setbacks. Recalls Chahal: 'In a multi-storey complex in Baliganagar, one of the pockets of Dharavi with a good sanitisation and social distancing facility, alarm bells rang on 5 April, when the virus found its way to one of the largest and most dense slums in the slum clusters of Dharavi—Mukund Nagar. Controlling the spread of the infection, given Mukund Nagar's crushing density, seemed almost impossible. The MCGM swung into action and within 48 hours barricaded the entry and exit points of the slum.

'We carried out the disinfection of 425 public toilets, began door-to-door screening and provided food packets to people during the world's strictest lockdown to slow down the spread of the pandemic in the slum. We classified every Covid-19 contact as high-risk, and over the next 2 months brought the situation under control. We built an environment of trust among the people, encouraging them to come out in the open and report their symptoms. Local doctors had a good rapport, built over several years, with the slum dwellers. It helped us control a virus that could have had catastrophic consequences in such a densely packed habitation.

'We set up 480 flu clinics across all the slums in Mumbai for people to come and give their swabs and get tested in. The civic body also took over some private hospitals so that it would have adequate treatment capacity. A steady decline in cases promoted the MCGM to consider an unlock plan for Dharavi. This included opening of small-scale industrial and pottery work units with minimum staff in July 2020. When the second UK-related Alpha mutant variant of the virus hit us in February 2021, we kept the manufacturing units in Dharavi humming. We did not want a repeat of the migrant labour exodus of the summer of 2020. Vaccination had begun and a lockdown would have caused more problems than it solved.'

Additional fever camps were set up to isolate non-Covid fever patients. The MCGM started announcing through vans regarding the location of fever camps to check symptoms of Covid-19. The civic body brought detection to the doorstep of the people. With testing in fever camps, high-risk contacts could be quickly shifted into quarantine. There was, in the early months, a trust deficit between the administration and slum residents. Many felt that the MCGM staff had come to the area only to evict them. Hence, the civic staff could not effectively screen, isolate and transfer patients to quarantine facilities.

Several hundred local medical practitioners worked as a bridge between the MCGM and the residents of Dharavi. People had faith in local doctors and followed their instructions diligently. At a private

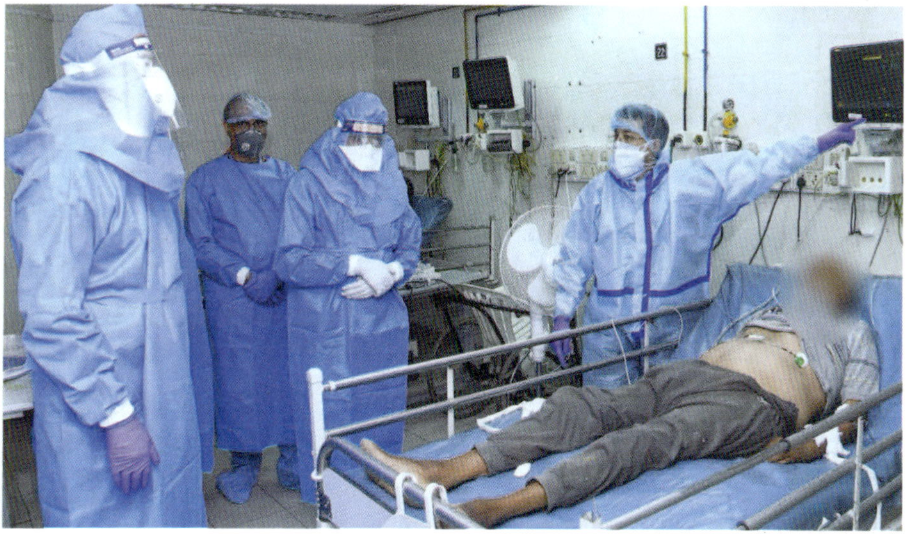

A Watershed Visit:
Chahal's first visit to Nair Hospital's Covid ICU on 9 May 2020, within a day of taking charge as municipal commissioner

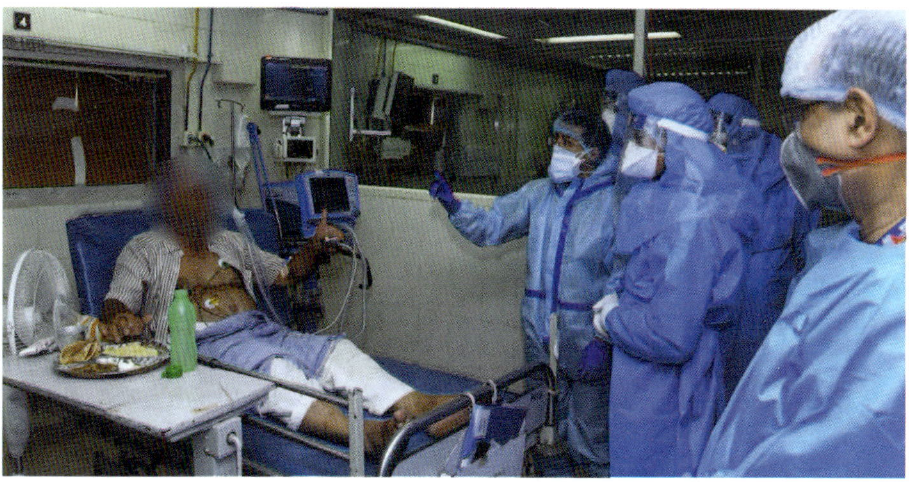

Receiving a briefing from senior doctors, after spending 53 minutes in the Covid ICU at Nair Hospital

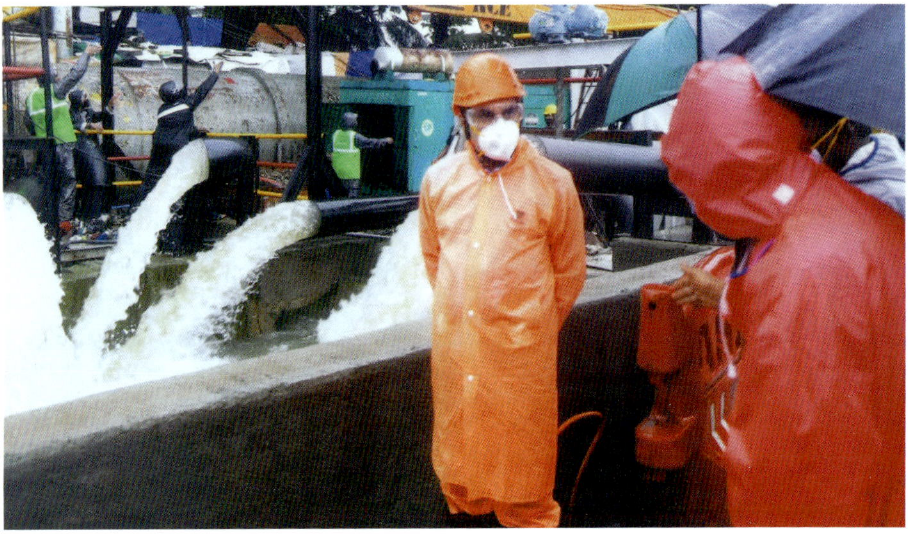

Chahal overseeing relief operations after the devastation caused by Cyclone Nisarga in Mumbai

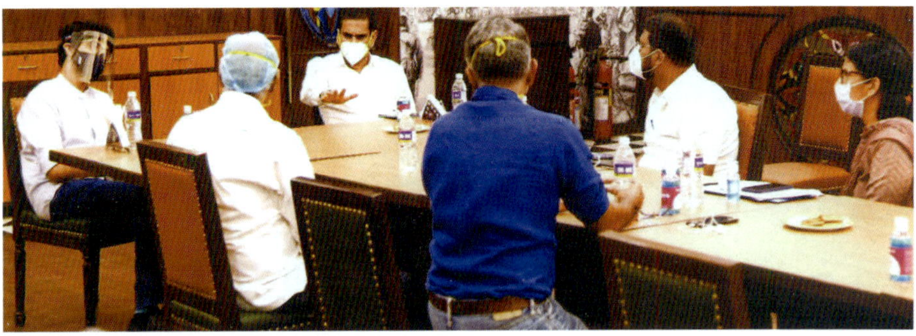

Leading the Way: Chahal briefs his team, along with Maharashtra's Environment Minister, Aaditya Thackeray, on 27 May 2020, when the Jumbo Dome at the NSCI in Worli was under construction

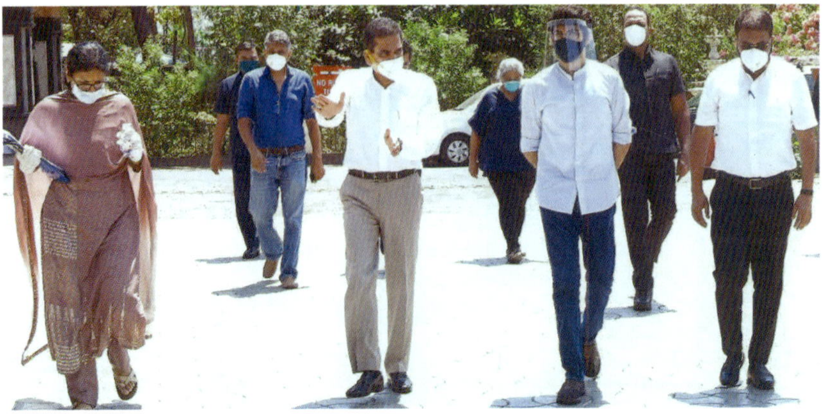

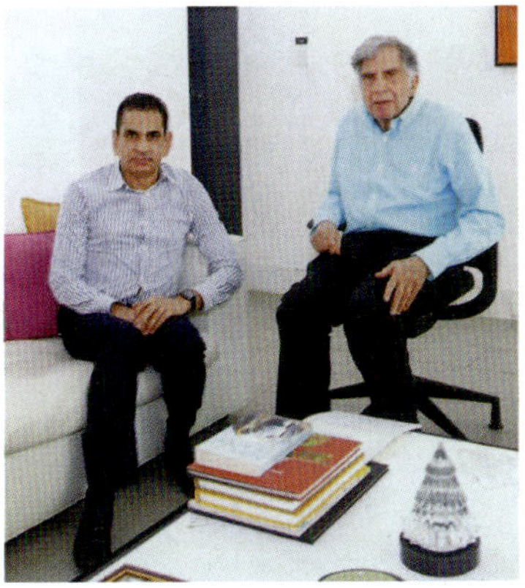

Chahal explaining the Mumbai Covid Fight Model to India's leading industrialist Ratan Tata at the latter's residence

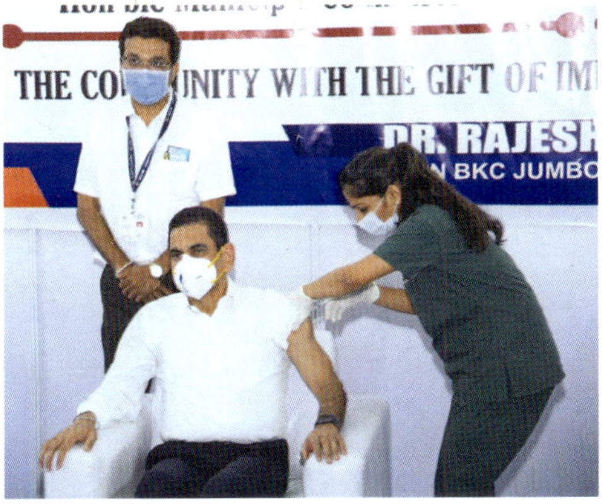

Chahal gets his vaccine jab

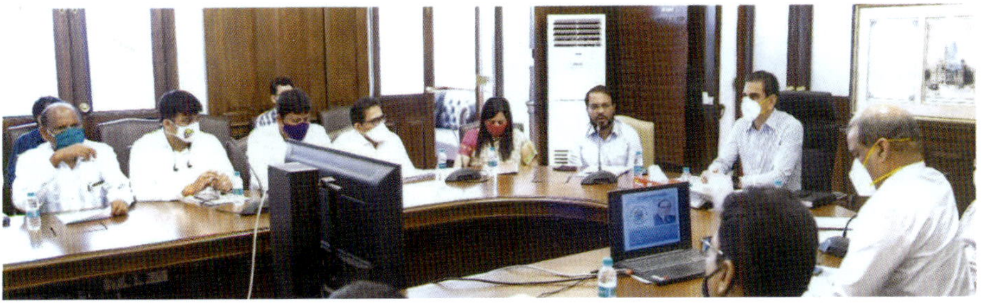

Chahal's Covid-19 review meeting with senior officers of the MCGM and Mumbai Police

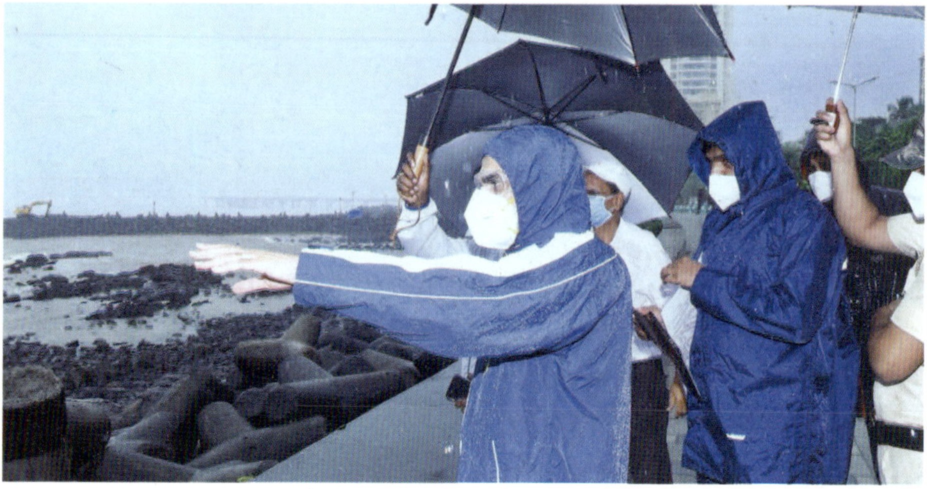

Field visits by Chahal and senior officers of MCGM during Cyclone Tauktae on 17 May 2021

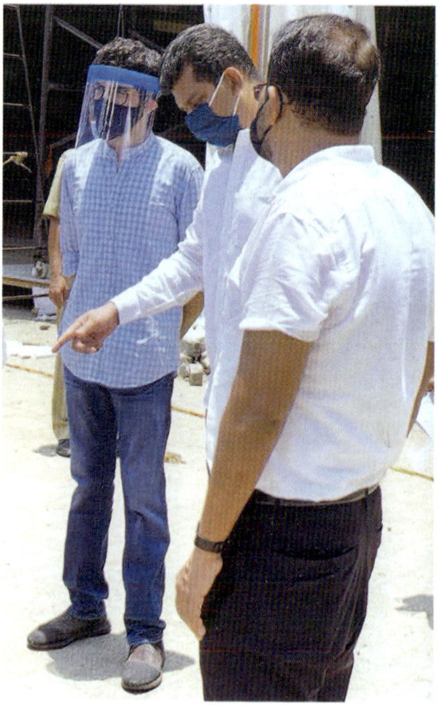

Visiting BKC Jumbo with Guardian Minister Aaditya Thackeray

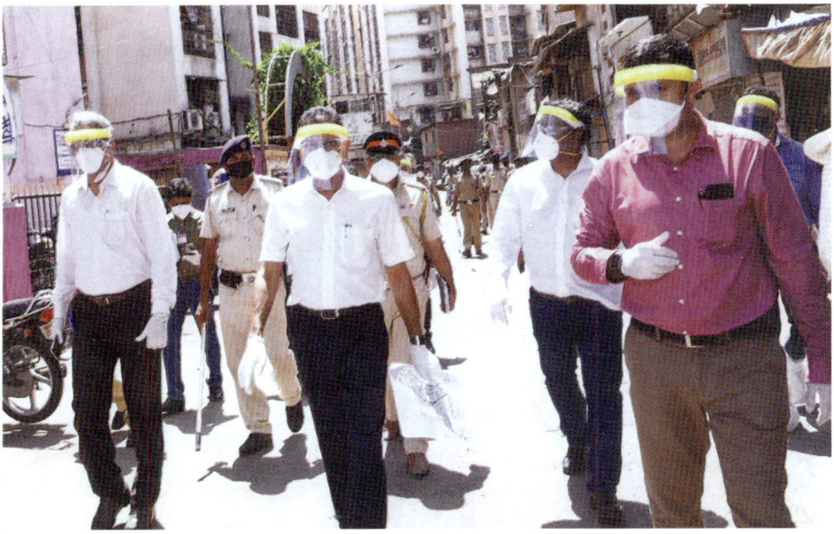

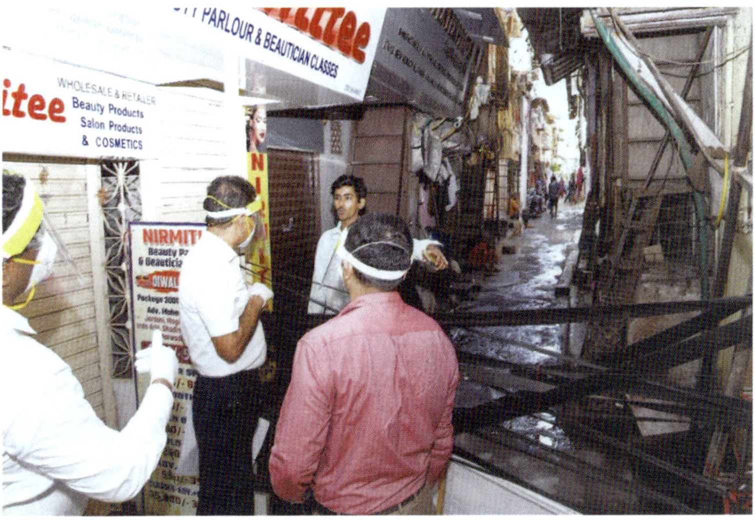

A march that set the tone for the 'chase the virus' strategy: Chahal leads his team of senior MCGM officers on a 5 km march in the Mukund Nagar Containment Zone of Dharavi on 9 May 2020, the very next day after being appointed the municipal commissioner, MCGM

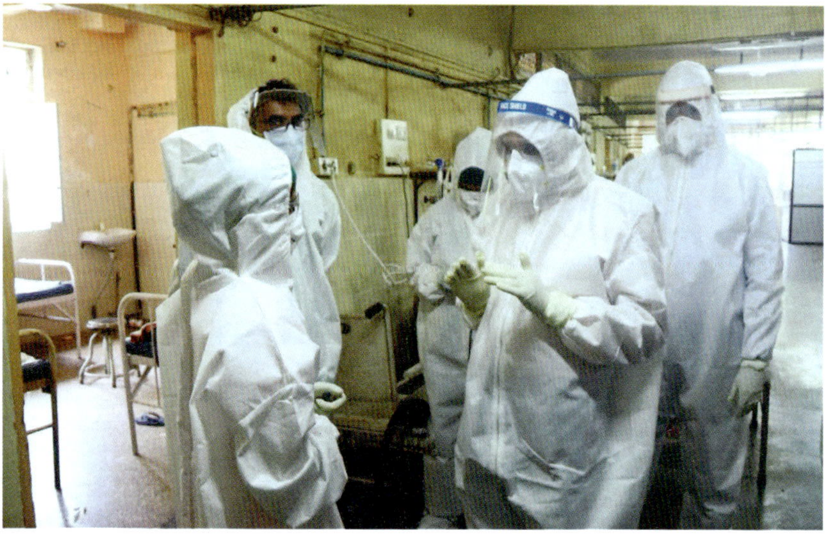

Being briefed by senior doctors during an hour-long visit to the Covid ICU at Sion Hospital on 17 May 2020, in the midst of the first wave

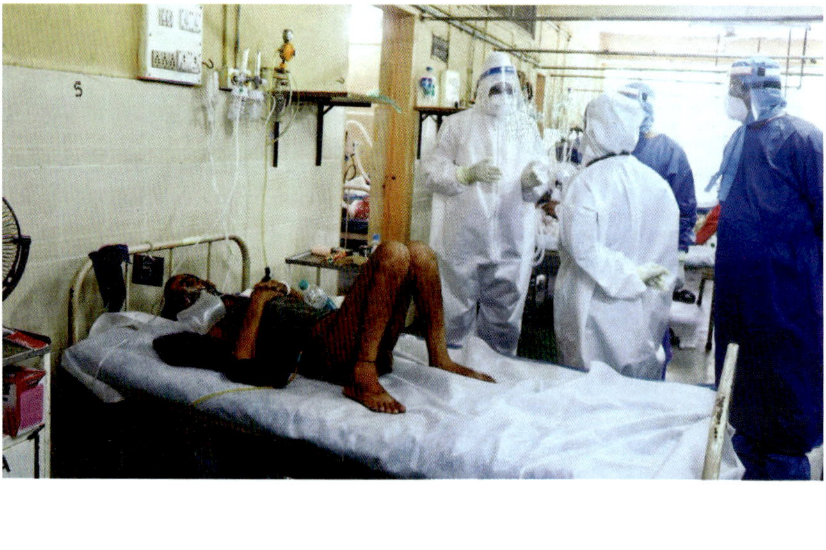

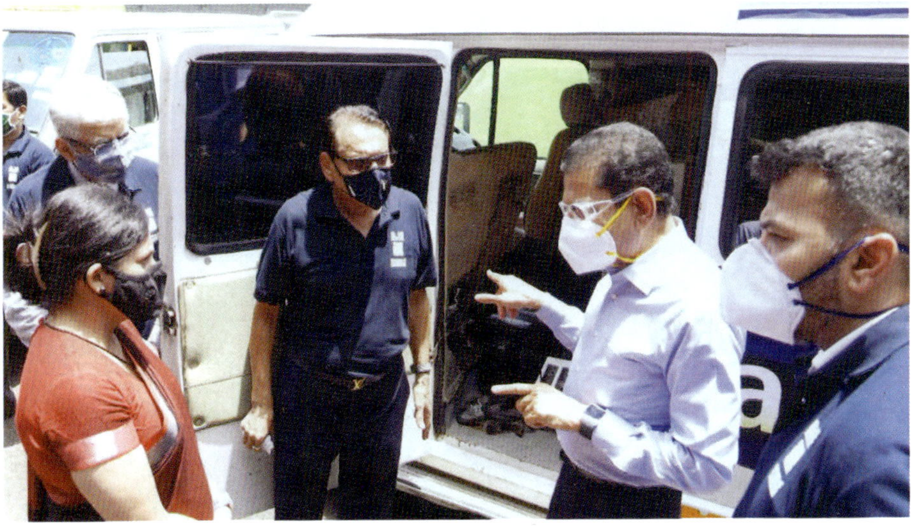

Launch of 'Mission Zero Covid' on 22 June 2020 at the Andheri Sports Complex, in collaboration with the NGO Bhartiya Jain Sanghatana and the Melinda Gates Foundation, in the presence of Shantilal Mehta and Ashwini Bhide, IAS

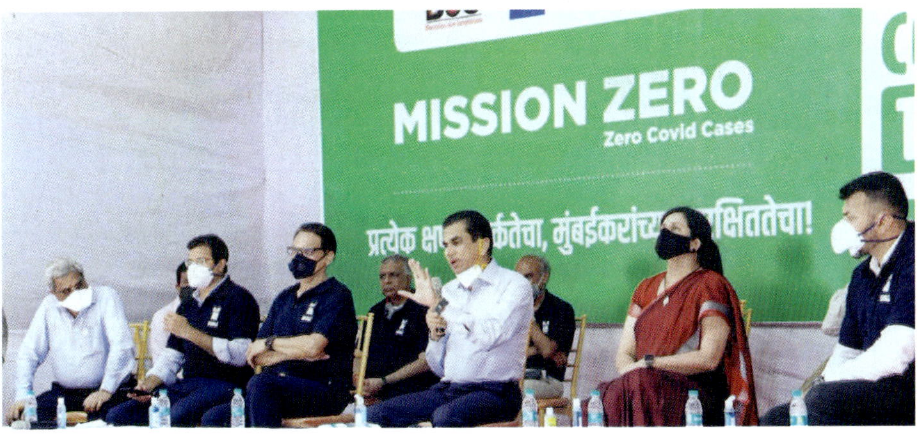

Delivering a briefing on 'Mission Zero Covid'

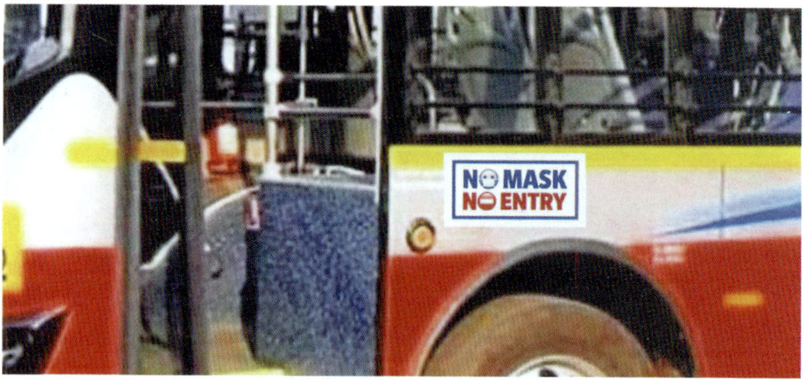

The MCGM's 'No Mask, No Entry' campaign on buses and taxis, as a part of the 'My Family, My Responsibility' initiative

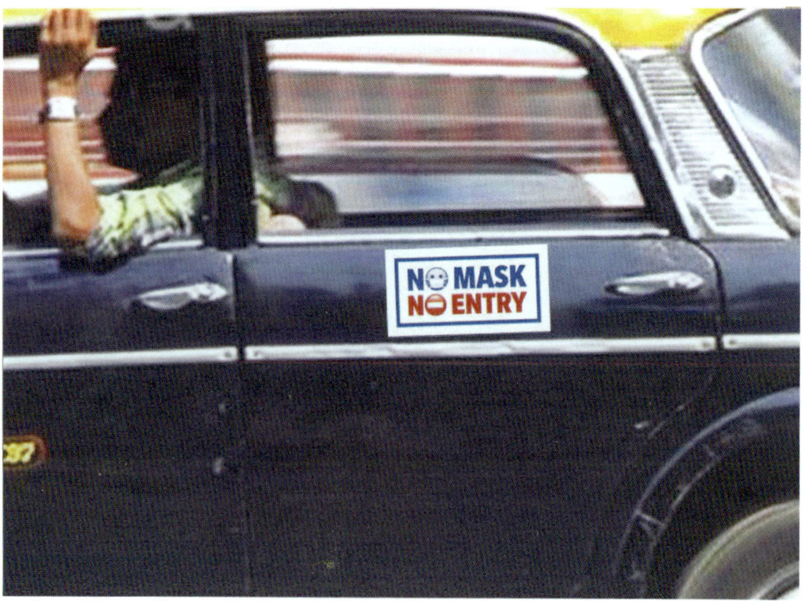

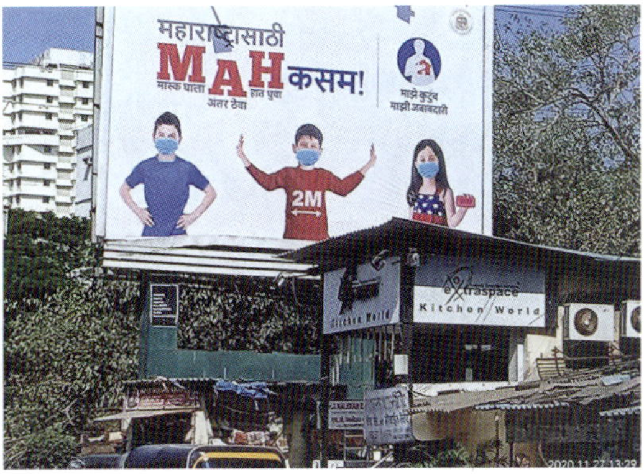

The MAH Kasam Campaign:
M = Mask;
A = Antar (Distancing);
H = Hand Sanitization,
in November–December, 2020

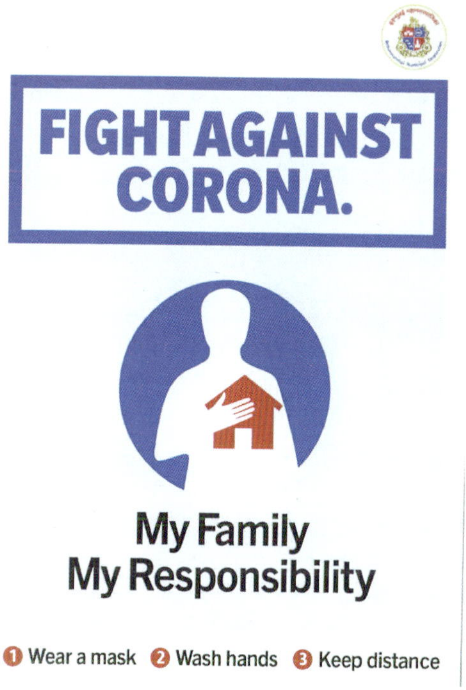

A series of outdoor campaigns helped raise awareness among citizens in Mumbai

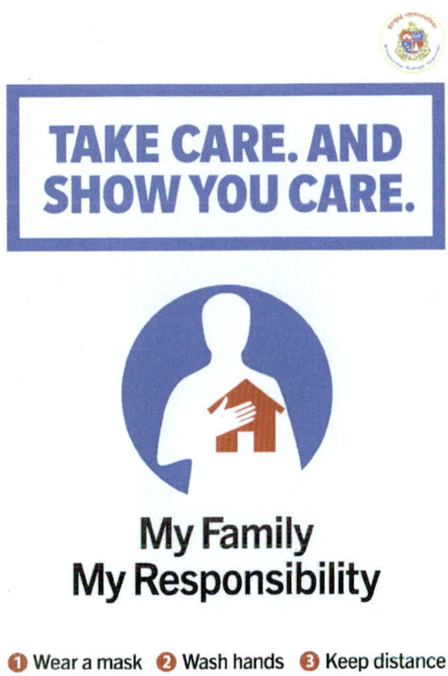

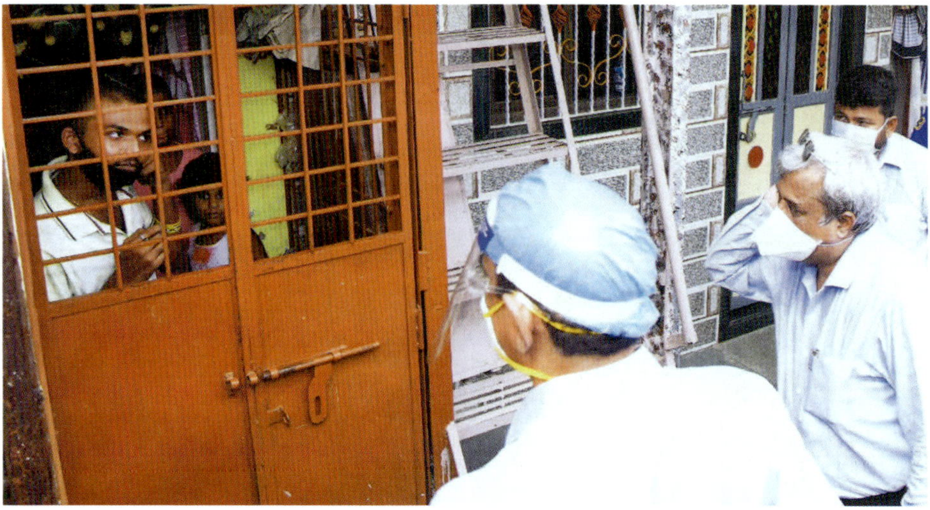

Chahal visits residents of the Appa Pada Containment Zone
in suburban Malad on 22 June 2020

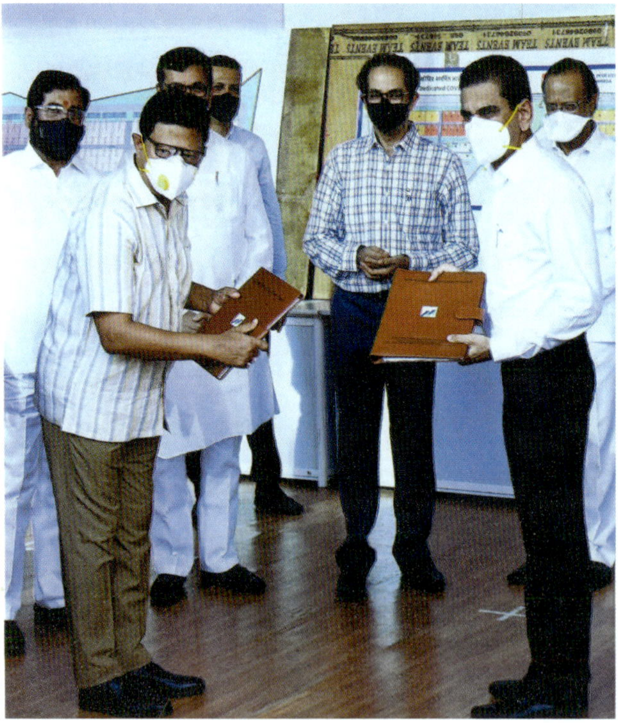

Handing over of BKC Jumbo from MMRDA to MCGM in the presence of
Chief Minister Uddhav Thackeray, Deputy Chief Minister Ajit Pawar
and Revenue Minister Balasaheb Thorat on 18 May 2020

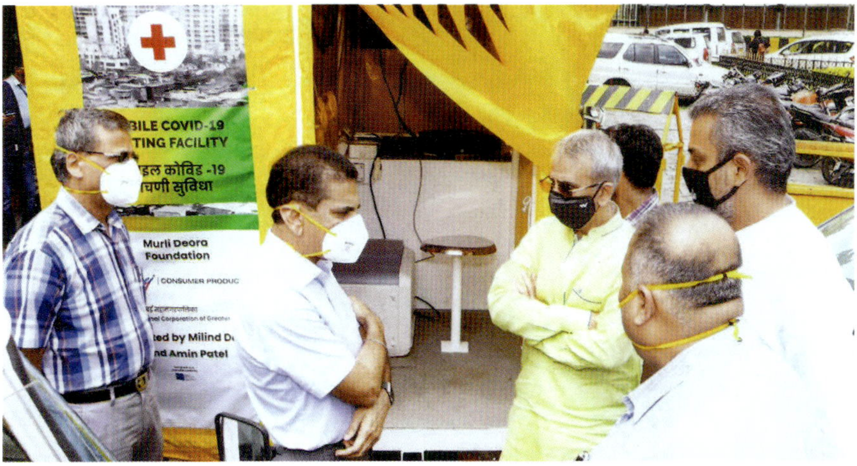

A mobile Covid test lab is donated to MCGM by Milind Deora and Amin Patel, MLA

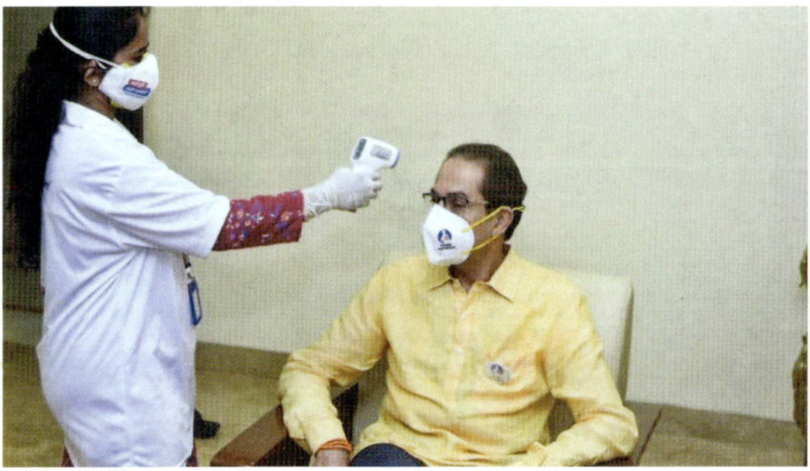

During the campaign, MCGM teams fanned out across Mumbai to personally visit and test every citizen, including Chief Minister Uddhav Thackeray, in their homes. Over 35.1 lakh families under MCGM's jurisdiction were visited, implying 99.1 per cent coverage

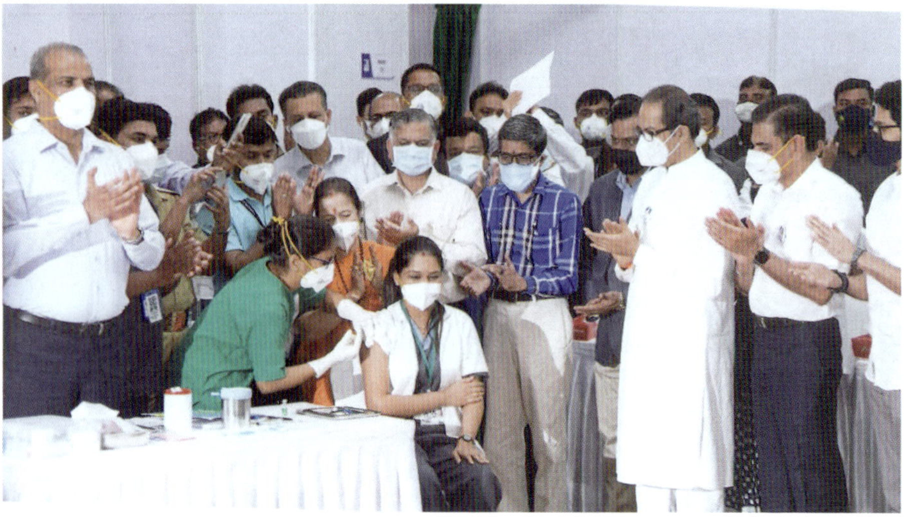

Launch of the National Vaccination Drive in Mumbai on 16 January 2021 at the hands of CM Uddhav Thackeray, in the presence of state government officials and state task force members at BKC Jumbo

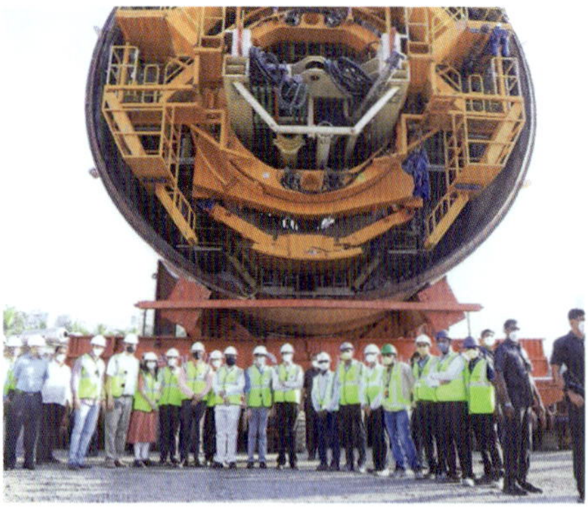

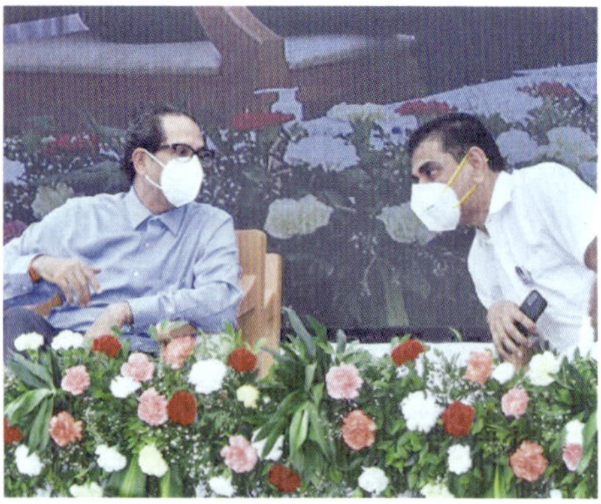

Launch of a 12.1-meter diameter tunnel boring machine under Malabar Hill by the Chief Minister, along with Chahal and Guardian Minister Aaditya Thackeray, on 11 January 2021, as a part of the Mumbai Coastal Road Project

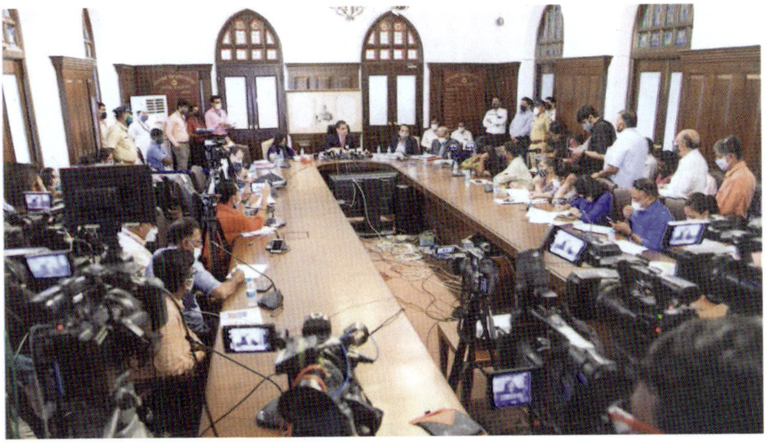

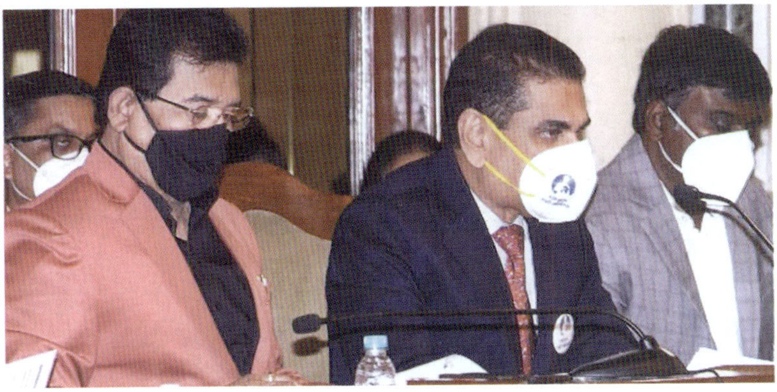

Chahal's 'Meet the Press' conference after the presentation of the MCGM Budget for 2021-2022 on 3 February 2021

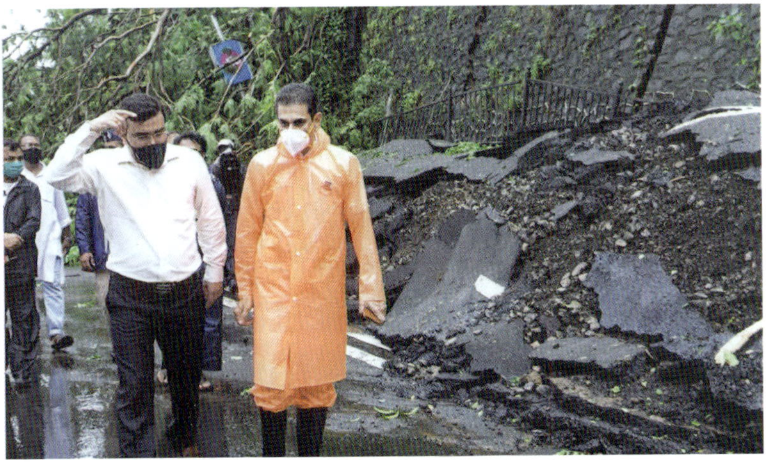

Inspecting the collapse of the Hanging Gardens' retaining wall, after a cloudburst and resultant flooding, along with the Ward Officer and senior Road Works officials

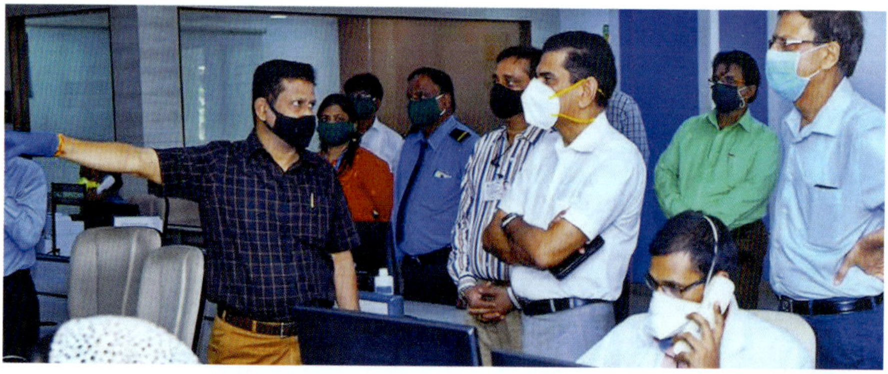

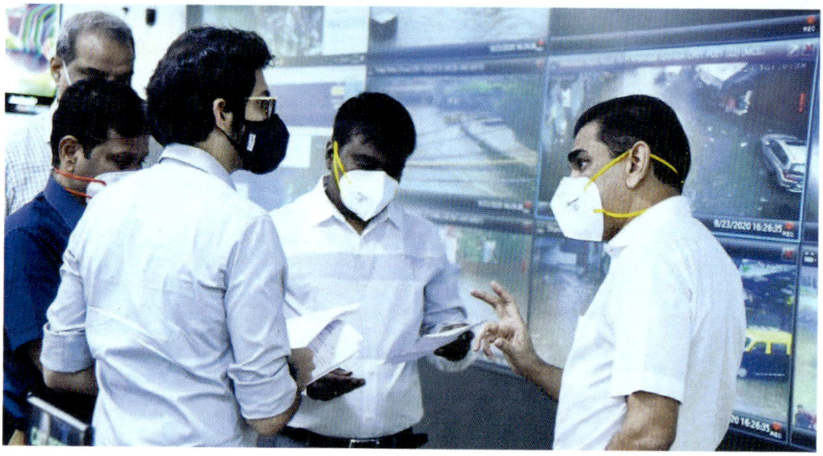

Preparatory meeting at MCGM's Disaster Control Room
in May 2021 to face Cyclone Tauktae

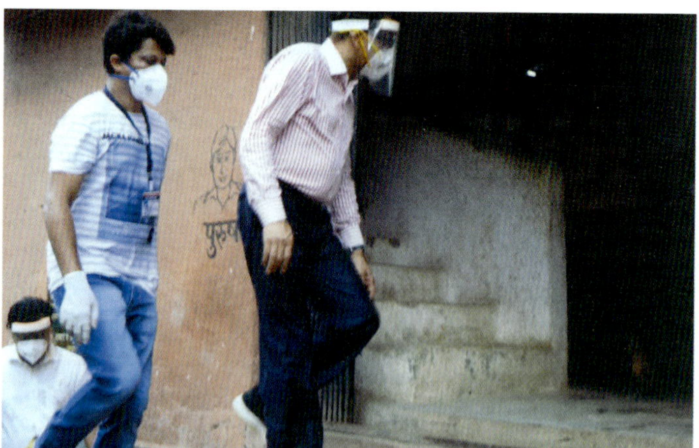

Chahal and his team inspect a public toilet in one of the hardest hit
Covid containment zones at Govandi in suburban Chembur

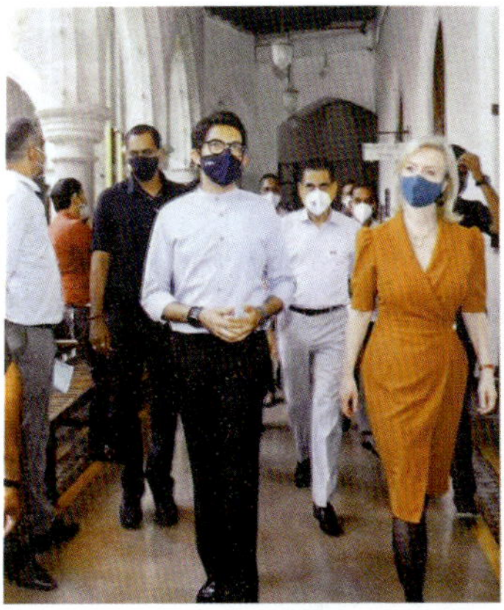

Elizabeth Truss, former Secretary of State for International Trade, UK, at the Municipal Commissioner's office on 9 February 2021

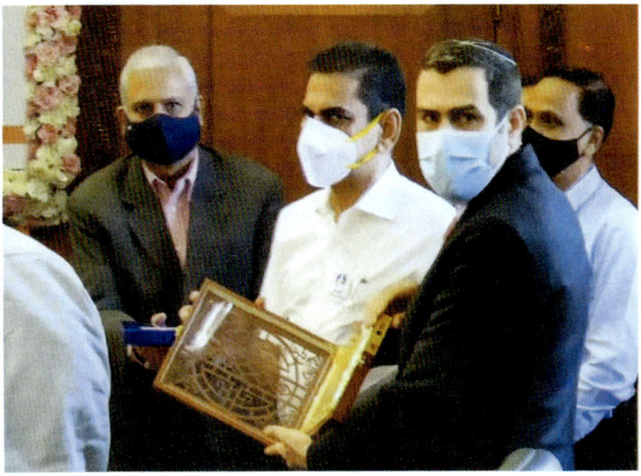

Signing of an MoU for the installation of the first desalination plant in Mumbai with the Consul General of Israel in Mumbai, Yaakov Finkelstein, and colleagues.

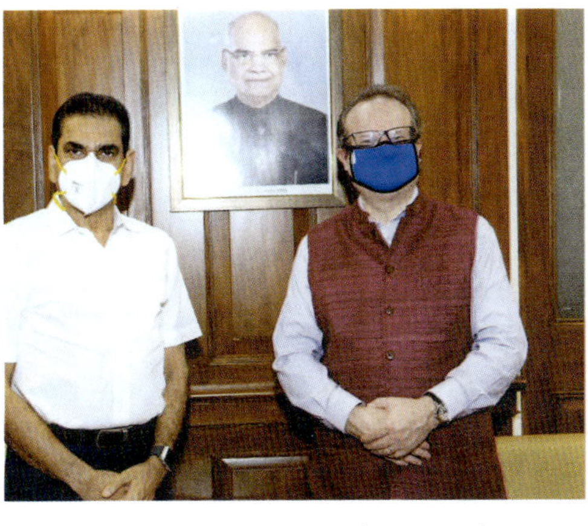

David Ranz, US Consul General in Mumbai, on a visit to Municipal Commissioner's office on 17 September 2020

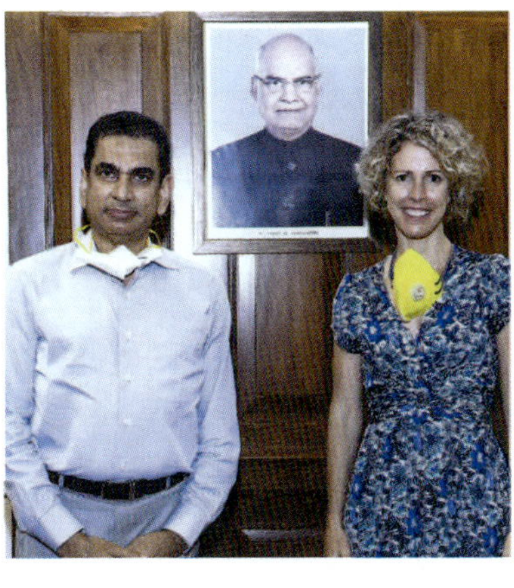

Sonia Babry, Consul General of France in Mumbai, at the Municipal Commissioner's office on 22 October 2020

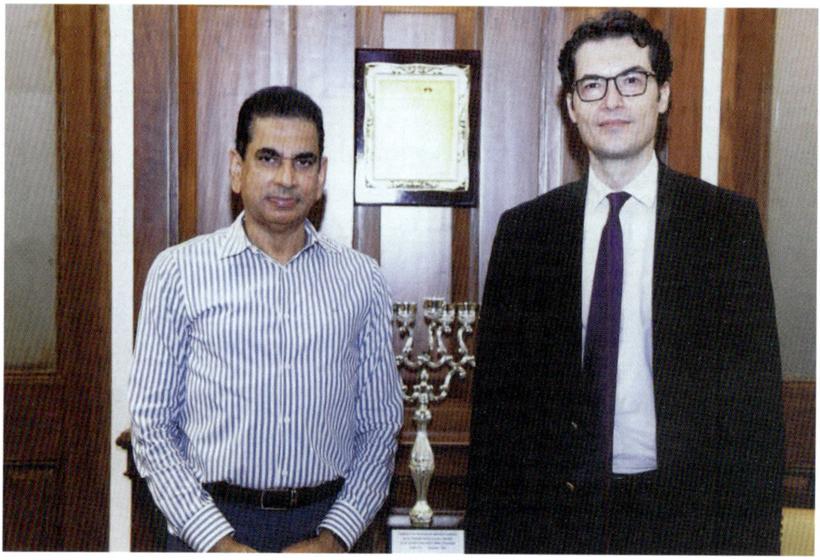

Ali Tolga Kaya, Consul General of Turkey, in the Municipal Commissioner's office on 31March 2021

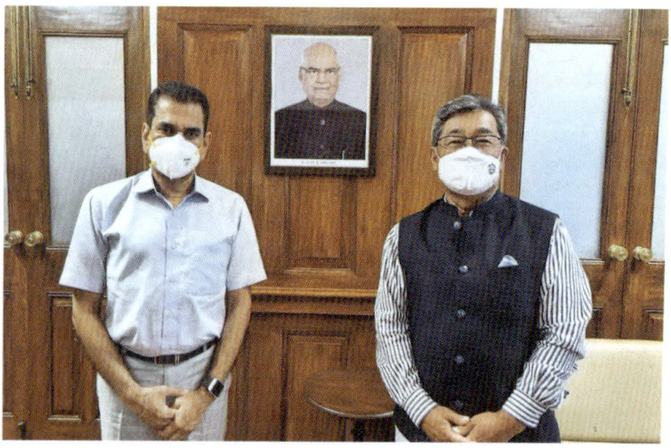

Chahal meets with Michio Haraoa, Consul General of Japan in Mumbai

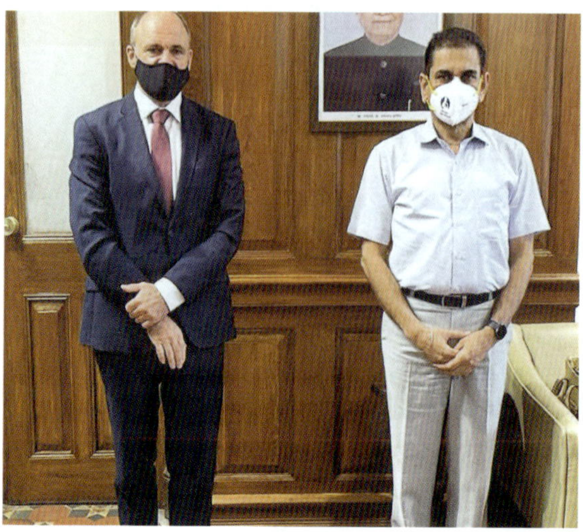

Bart De Jons, Consul General of the Netherlands with Chahal

Inspecting pre-monsoon preparations and desilting of the Mithi river

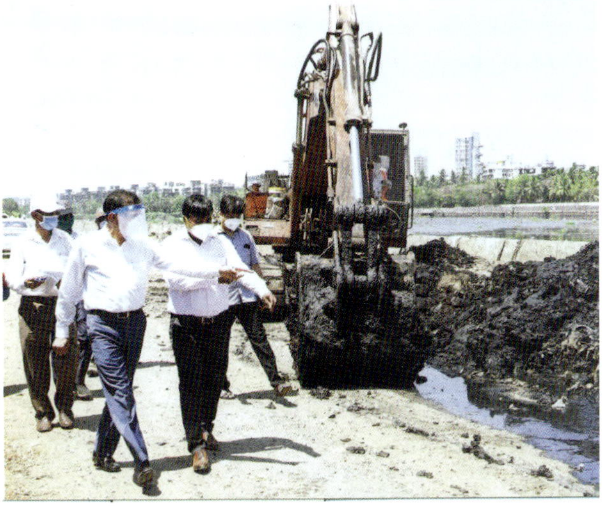

Chief Justice of the Bombay High Court, Dipankar Datta, felicitates Chahal on 14 May 2021 for successful Covid management

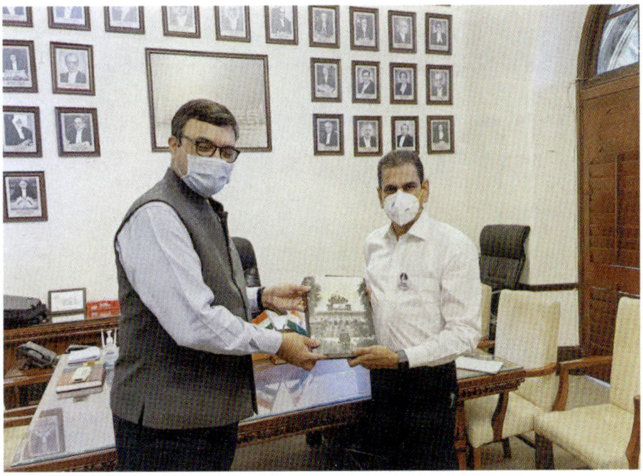

Inauguration of the Heritage Walk to MCGM's HQ, in the presence of the CM, Deputy CM, Revenue Minister, Environment Minister and the Mayor, on Republic Day, 26 January 2021

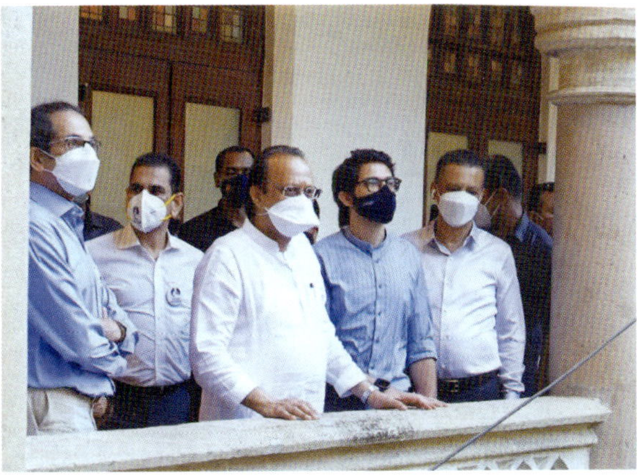

A hilarious, but very apt Tweet by the well-known Pune based cartoonist Alok on 7 May 2021

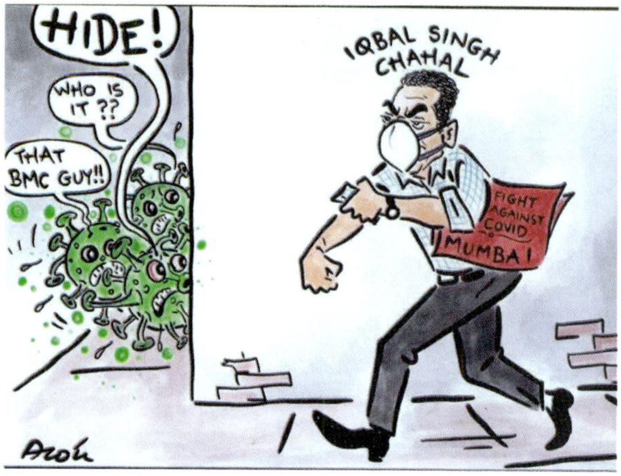

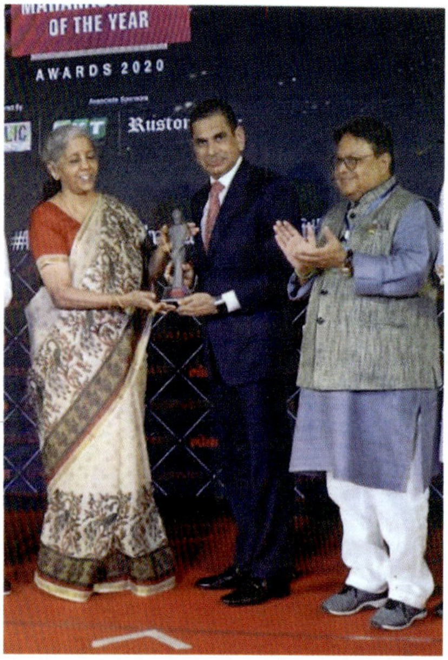

Chahal receiving the *Maharashtrian of the Year 2021* award from Nirmala Sitharaman, Union Minister for Finance, at a special ceremony in New Delhi

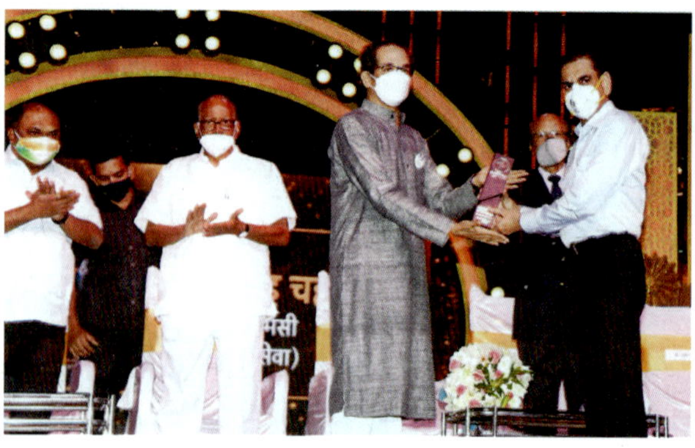

CM Uddhav Thackeray hands over the *Sakaal Samman Award 2021* in the presence of veteran NCP leader Sharad Pawar

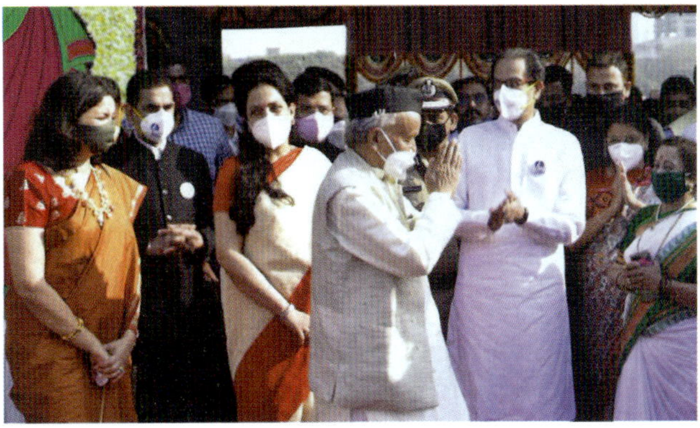

With Maharashtra Governor BS Koshyari, CM Thackeray and his wife Rashmi and the Mayor of Mumbai, Kishori Pednekar, during the ceremony for the *Mumbai Ratna 2021* award presented to Chahal

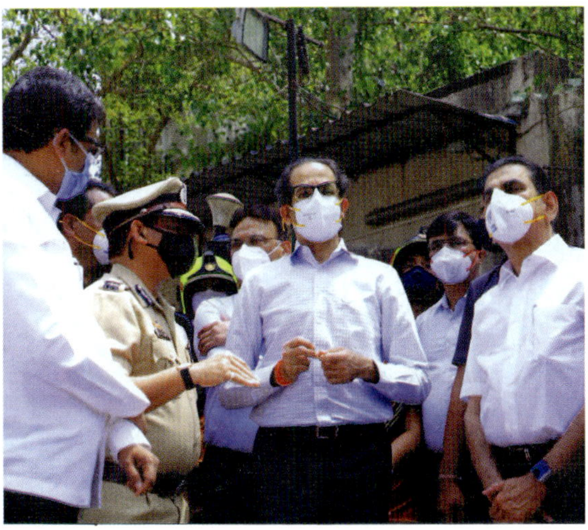

Briefing the CM at one of many field visits during the peak of the pandemic in Mumbai

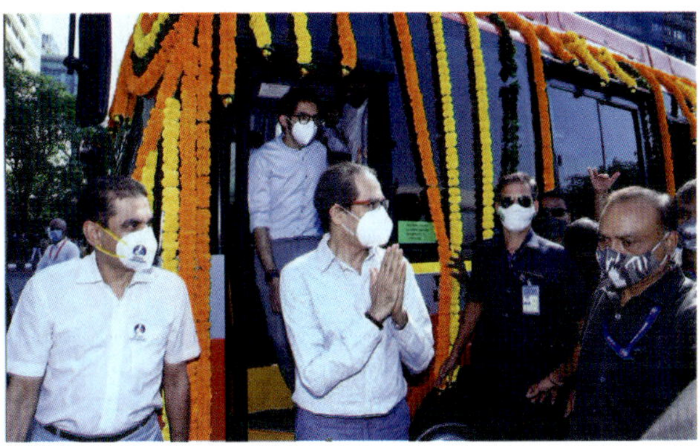

Introduction of electric buses by BEST in Mumbai

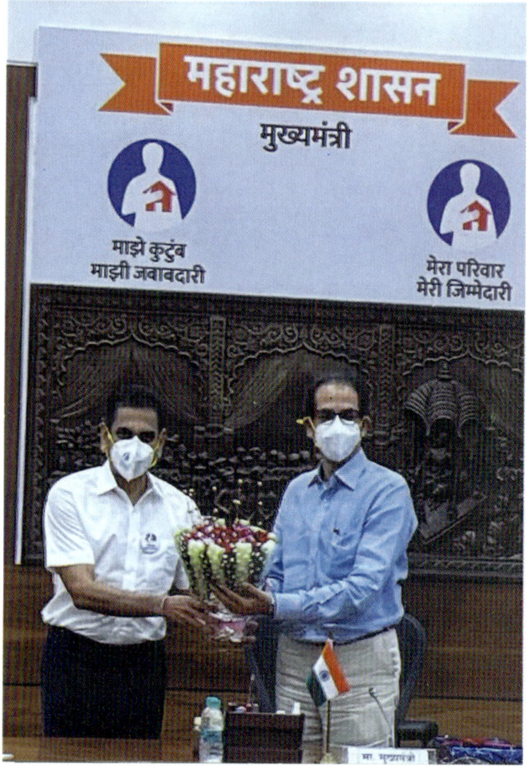

Release of the *MCGM Covid Manual* at the hands of the CM

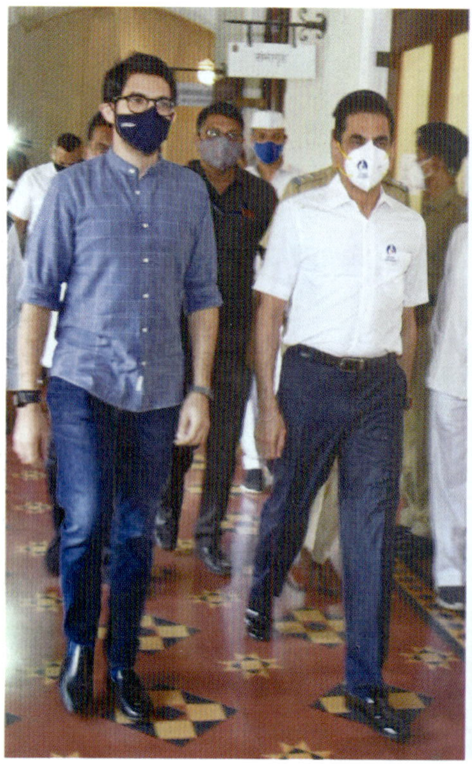

Heading for a Covid review meeting at MCGM's HQ, accompanied by Aaditya Thackeray, in November 2020

Arriving to attend a formal function on Independence Day, 15 August 2020

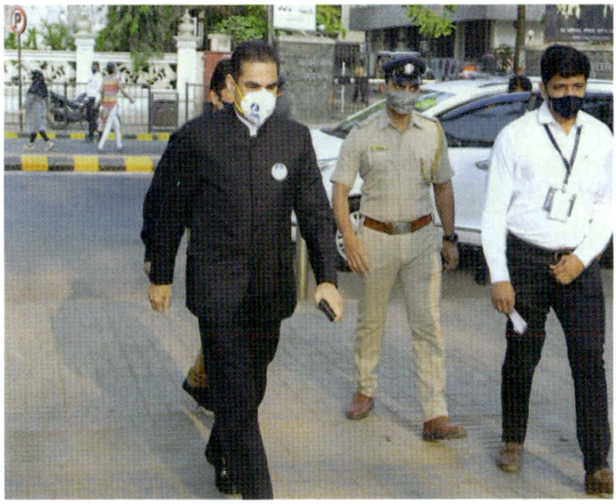

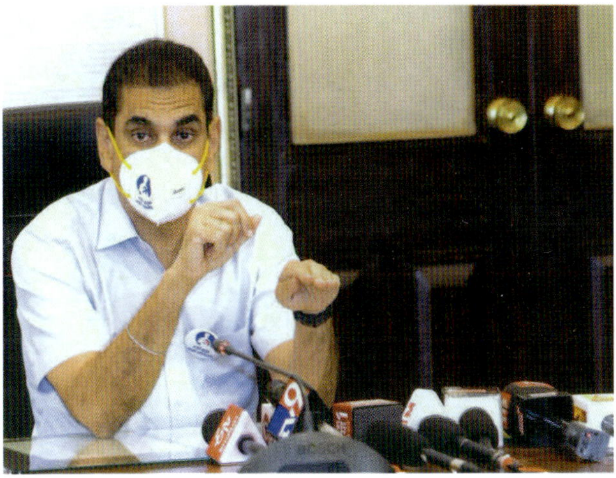

Conducting a media briefing on Covid in January 2021

Ceremonial breaking of a coconut on the arrival of the first consignment of Covishield vaccine in Mumbai on 31 January 2021

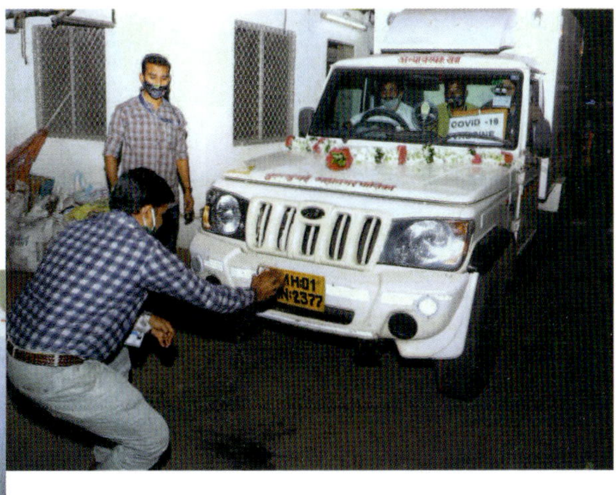

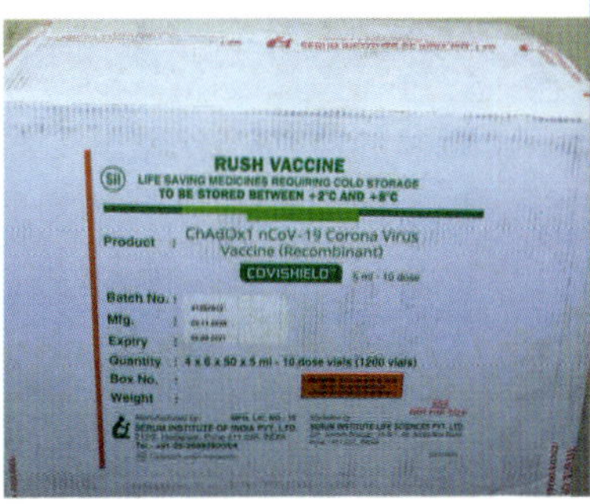

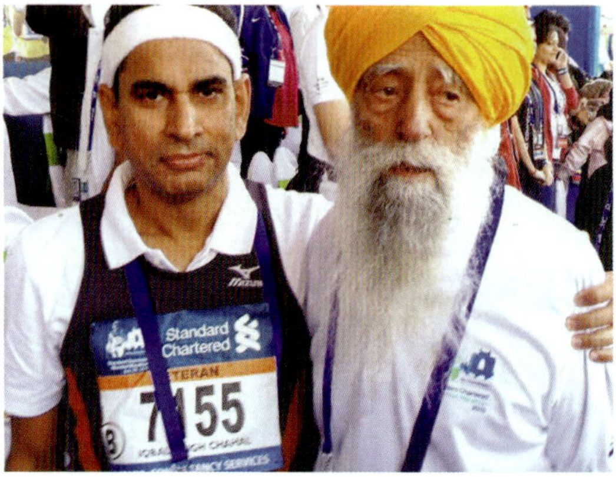

With the 104-year-old Fauja Singh from the UK, who ran in the Standard Chartered Half-Marathon in 2013

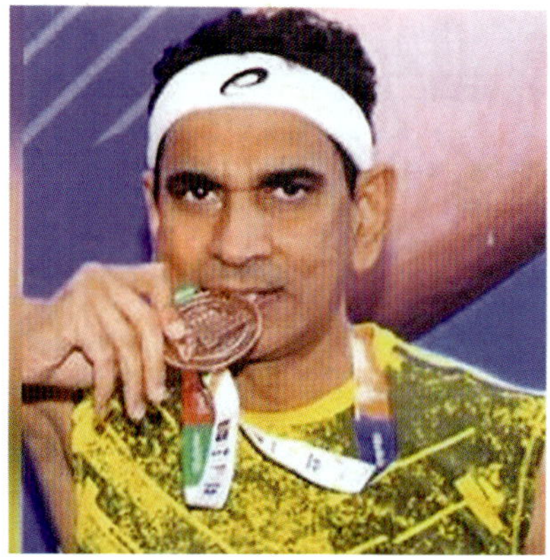

Chahal, a fitness enthusiast and an avid yoga practitioner, has competed in 17 half-marathons in Mumbai since 2004, including the Tata Mumbai Half-Marathon, held in January 2020, shortly before the Covid pandemic struck

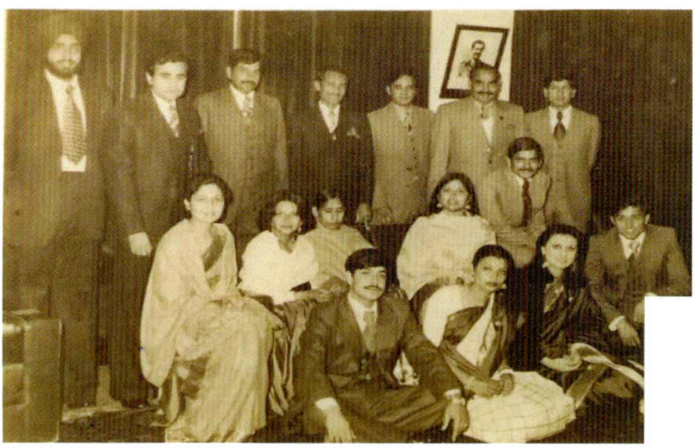

Chahal's father, Colonel Man Singh Chahal (Retd.), pictured in the 16th Light Cavalry Regiment Mess in 1978 (*last row, standing second from right, with moustache*), and Chahal's mother Gurdev Kaur Chahal (*second row, sitting second from left*)

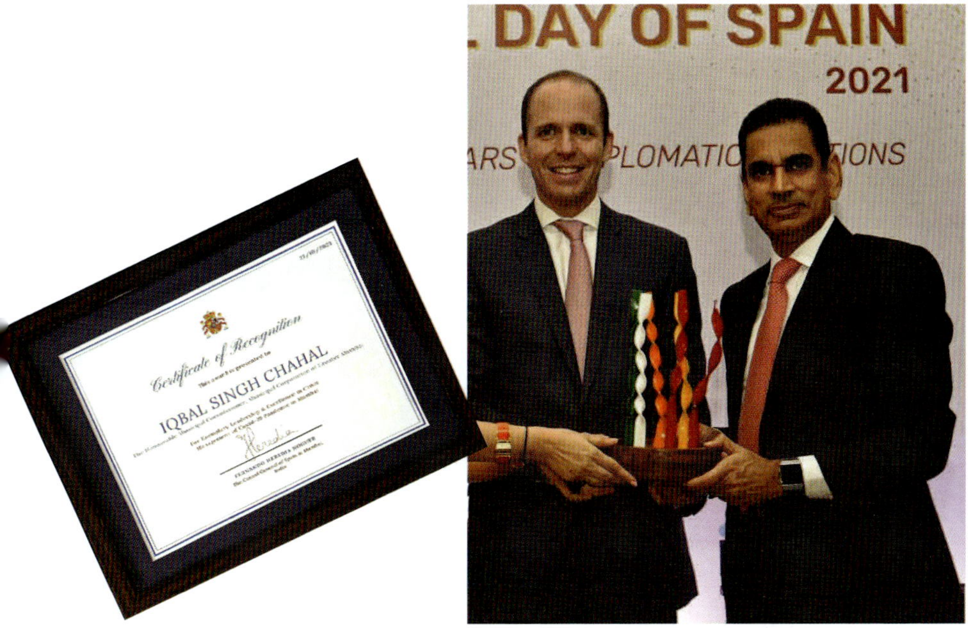

Receiving the *Certificate of Recognition* awarded by the Kingdom of Spain, at the hands of Fernando Heredia, Spain's Consul General in Mumbai, on 27 October 2021, for exemplary leadership and excellence in crisis management of the Covid-19 pandemic

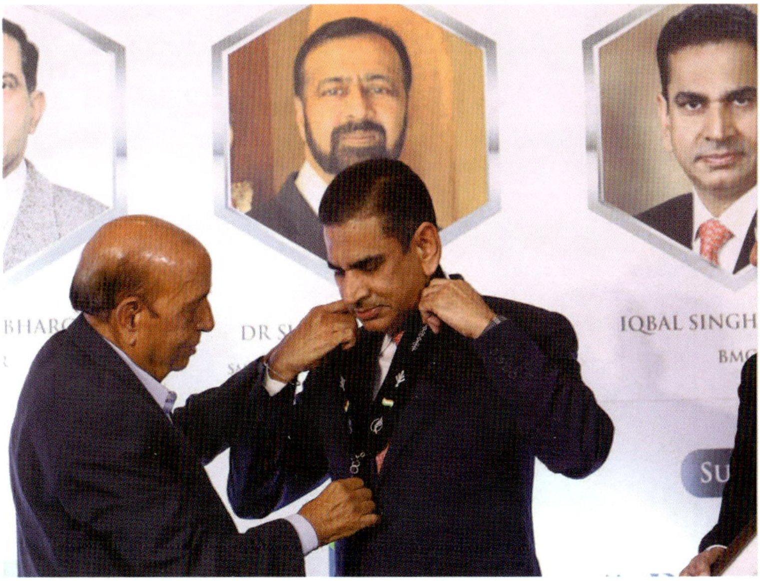

Chahal receiving the QIMPRO award and QIMPRO medal on 16 November 2021 for extraordinary achievement in a unique space (Covid pandemic management in Mumbai). The QIMPRO award is not an annual award and has been presented only on four occasions in the past 30 years

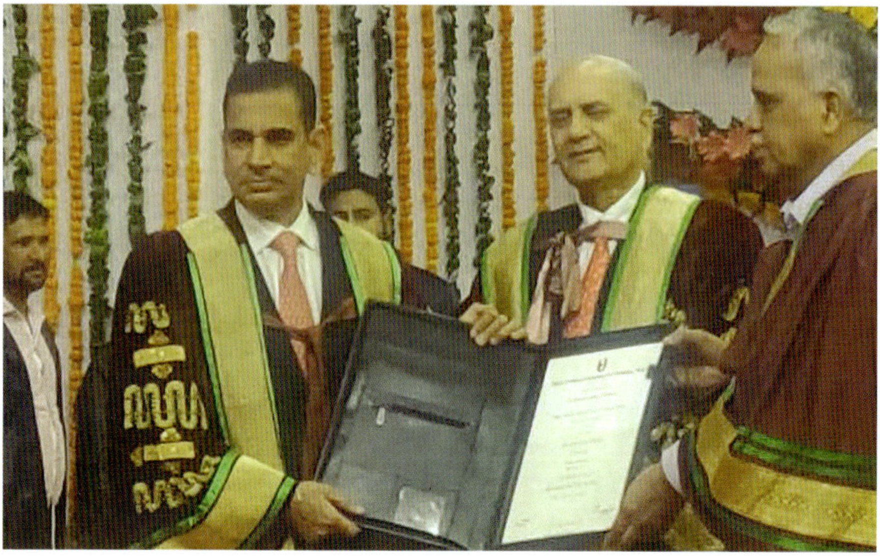

Chahal receiving an honorary 'Doctor of Science' degree (*Honoris Causa*) for his stellar performance in management of the Covid pandemic, from his alma mater, Thapar Institute of Engineering and Technology (deemed to be a university), in Patiala, Punjab, at a special convocation held on 8 November 2021

Thapar Institute of Engineering and Technology, Patiala

(Deemed-to-be-University)

This is to make known that

the Senate and the Board of Governors

of

Thapar Institute of Engineering and Technology, Patiala

assembled in the 35th Convocation

held on 8th November, 2021

have conferred upon

Shri Iqbal Singh Chahal

the Degree of

Doctor of Science

(Honoris Causa)

under Clause 4(xliv) of the

Memorandum of Association, June 2007

Given under the seal of the Institute

Registrar

Director

Chairman Board of Governors

doctor's clinic in Dharavi, this approach yielded dividends. Local authorities were able to screen people, including senior citizens, who were most vulnerable. The MCGM screened residents in a short period of time by going house-to-house. Since patients were screened and isolated early, they could be continuously monitored, avoiding a rise in the mortality rate.

'Whatever the final outcome,' Chahal says, 'Dharavi has been a great success story. It is integral to the success of the Mumbai Model. In Dharavi, we did not wait for a vaccine to come, we did not wait for medicines like Remdesivir to be introduced. It was basically batting on the front foot, setting up a system, going from home to home for surveillance, checking the oxygen levels of people, checking temperatures, and putting high-risk contacts into local dharamshalas or quarantining them in hotels. Surveillance was a key factor in the success of both the Dharavi and Mumbai models. Community leaders, played a very critical role. An equally critical role was played by the private medical practitioners and the NGOs who acted as a link between the MCGM health officials and the local people.

'Even today, we remain vigilant in these vulnerable areas to protect them from future waves or surges. If the feedback we get is negative, the MOH (medical officer of health) is alerted. Each ward is headed by an MOH. The MOH has a team of several hundred people across health and administrative domains. They can monitor which MCGM team visited which containment zone and when.'

Over 2020 and 2021, the corporation suspended several workers who were missing in action. The MCGM's healthcare workers are paid well—over ₹60,000 a month. They were expected to perform as per the protocol that had been laid down. The ward war room teachers passed on information to the MOH or ward war room officer. If food packs were of poor quality, the message went to the ward officer. If a surveillance team was missing in action, the feedback was again conveyed to the MOH. Immediate corrective steps were taken.

Chahal adds another task that was undertaken in this overall strategy. 'We had to keep the entire slum environment clean—not just the toilets, but also the lanes, bylanes, garbage collection centres and gutters,' he says. 'We ensured the sanitisation of lanes and bylanes and checked whether waste disposal was being done properly or not. Our task focused on young boys in the slums who would be constantly moving in and out, increasing the possibility of spreading the infection. The police had sealed several lanes and bylanes, but if there was still too much movement of people in and out of the slums or the containment zones, we asked for additional police deployment there. In many places where the crowd was aggressive, we asked the police commissioner to deploy armed state reserve police (SRP). The feedback on this also came to us from the community leaders.

'The final task was very important: we told our community leaders that if they had a population of 4,000 under them, the number of elderly people would be small. So we decided to start giving an honorarium of ₹10,000 a month to the community leader. We directed him to make house-to-house visits and check if the elderly people in that particular family were being taken care of. Depending on their feedback, we would dispatch an ambulance and our workers would pick up the patient and place him in a Covid Care Centre. In Dharavi, we placed 50 mobile dispensaries which were given to us by philanthropist Shantilal Mutha and funded by the Melinda and Bill Gates Foundation. The job of the community leaders was to ensure that if our healthcare workers, through an oversight, left any person unattended, they must inform us so that our team could pick him up and either treat him in a mobile dispensary or admit him to a hospital.

'These key functions were unique to the community leaders in Mumbai's containment zones. The system was not in place anywhere else in the country. And it has proved to be a game changer in the slums, chawls, tenements and other containment zones in the city right through these 2 years of the Covid-19 pandemic. Our surveillance system helped identify and treat people with early Covid symptoms. The death rate fell. More and more people started getting picked up faster and treated sooner. Doctors in their slum clinics began treating non-Covid illnesses too. The suppppliers of food packets also became vigilant because they knew they would be caught in the net for supplying poor quality food.

'At the time we did not have a vaccine. But the concept of community leaders and real-time feedback moved matters in the right direction. We were an army of people doing the job on ground zero. The MCGM has access to ample funds, apart from the power to impose restrictions when and where needed. This will be a key mitigating factor in subsequent waves triggered by new variants of the coronavirus in the months ahead in 2022 and beyond.'

The MCGM had recognised early the crucial role that testing would play in combating—and overcoming—the Covid-19 pandemic. Displaying prescience, the civic body on 23 June 2020, issued this official note: 'The MCGM's all-round efforts to limit the spread of the coronavirus are showing promising results. In line with its aggressive approach in the city's fight against the virus, the MCGM has now launched Mission Universal Testing. The most important component of this mission is the MCGM's decision to procure 1 lakh antigen testing kits that provide reports in less than half an hour. Corporate houses and private companies too, have been advised to test their employees by purchasing rapid testing kits. In the presence of Municipal Commissioner Iqbal Singh Chahal, a meeting of various additional municipal commissioners, concerned joint commissioners, deputy commissioners, assistant commissioners and chief executive officers of various medical laboratories was held on 23 June 2020 via video conferencing, where the Municipal Commissioner gave a host of instructions to all the concerned officials. Mission Universal Testing aims to trace, test and provide timely treatment to citizens in order to control the spread of the virus. All of these measures will play an important role in helping the city to achieve that goal.'

As winter descended over Mumbai in December 2020, the city breathed again. Cases and deaths had moderated. The first wave of the pandemic seemed to have waned. The *Indian Express* and the *New Indian Express* invited Chahal to assess how the city had coped so far with Covid-19. In his op-ed published on 4 December 2020, Chahal described the battle Mumbai had fought against the pandemic for the past 9 months. The op-ed encapsulated the extraordinary crisis Mumbai had faced and seemingly overcome—for the moment:

> 'Ever since the first Covid case was detected in Mumbai in mid-March 2020, the city got into the news for all the wrong reasons. It appeared that the offensive march of Covid was relentless. The pandemic spread like wildfire in the months of March and April. The well-known slums of Mumbai like Dharavi, Deonar, Bainganwadi, Govandi, Ghatkopar and Worli-Koliwada were on fire. The death rate touched 8 per cent of cases detected, and it was speculated that the city would see innumerable deaths.
>
> 'In the first week of May, a few bodies were seen on the streets and road dividers. The situation seemed visibly out of control. Social media was flooded with videos of bodies on the road and stacked in public hospitals next to patients undergoing treatment. The Government of India's Covid Monitoring Team visited Mumbai on 5 May, expressing fears that there was mismanagement and the infection was likely to explode leading to thousands of fatalities. Some critics even raised the demand of handing over Mumbai to the army.
>
> 'Panic gripped the city as it became the country's most-talked-about hotspot. It was in this scenario that I took over on 8 May

as Mumbai's municipal commissioner. Early morning, on the very next day, I walked into the Covid ICUs of the municipal hospitals to take stock of the desperate ground reality; and we followed it up with a march through the containment zones of Dharavi to understand the situation prevailing in the slums.

'From first-hand experience, we identified four pillars on which the Covid fight would stand: testing discipline, need of ambulances, ensuring availability of Covid beds, and an abundant number of trained doctors/paramedics. The focus was on testing, tracing, tracking, quarantine and treatment. In the next 10 weeks, the Municipal Corporation of Greater Mumbai (MCGM) ensured a multifold increase in the city's health infrastructure.

'It was made mandatory that Covid test results would be available within 24 hours. Thousands of health workers entered the slums and containment zones for door-to-door surveillance and focused testing. There was a tenfold increase in ambulances from 80 to 826, and these were at hand by making them accessible on the Uber platform and on-call free of cost. More than 1,000 doctors and paramedics were hired under the banner of "Covid Warriors" from among retired government doctors.

'Around 900 intern MBBS students were deployed to manage the 24-hour war rooms, one in each municipal ward, fully equipped with ambulances, doctors and paramedics round the clock. The Covid fight was decentralised with each of the 24 wards of Mumbai acting independently. An innovative and extremely aggressive chase the virus policy was implemented effectively and lakhs of high-risk contacts were physically shifted from the slums and put in institutional quarantine zones to prevent spread and to disconnect them from the virus.

'A world-class online platform for dialysis management for

Covid patients was implemented. Mumbai was the first city to set up centrally air-conditioned Jumbo field hospitals with ICU and dialysis beds; walk-in facilities of beds for suspected Covid patients were created all over the city to treat suspected patients without test reports; and dashboards were created for hospitals to monitor the crematorium status.

'For hospitalised patients, Mission Save Lives was successfully implemented to reduce the mortality rate to under 2 per cent from the earlier 8 per cent; and a compensation of ₹50 lakh was provided for deceased municipal and BEST transport staff not covered under the Government of India Insurance Scheme. The outreach programme too worked wonders. The "My Family My Responsibility" campaign was implemented for 2 months where more than 12,000 healthcare workers reached out to 3.5 million families to ensure health check-ups.

'The city was painted red with the slogan 'No-Mask-No-Entry' on thousands of hoardings and bus stops, buses and taxis. The campaign also included a deterrent and more than 5 lakh people were fined for not wearing masks. iPads with WiFi facilities were distributed to admitted Covid-positive patients for interaction with their relatives. Team MCGM has risen to the occasion. We can take heart that the city has arrested the pandemic, making Mumbai one of the safest metropolises in the country. But there is no room for complacency as the war against Covid-19 is far from over.'

Within 2 months, Chahal's warning proved prophetic as a second wave of Covid-19 swept through the city in February 2021. Battle was rejoined. The second wave of the pandemic in 2021 quickly took daily cases across India back to nearly 1,00,000—a level seen at the peak of the first wave. In a matter of weeks, cases rose to over 4,00,000 a day, among the highest in the world. Mumbai recorded over 11,000 cases—the highest ever for the city—on 4 April 2021. Chahal doubled testing in Mumbai. Logistical problems on account of a limited lockdown in Mumbai made the number of tests wobble up and down, but the intent was clear: *chase the virus*.

'The best strategy to defeat the virus is to chase the virus,' Chahal declares. 'Because if you catch the virus early, then deaths are minimised. In the second wave in 2021, 85 per cent of the cases were asymptomatic. Existing SOPs were tightly implemented. People not wearing masks were fined and given masks to put on. If guests at a marriage function numbered more than 50, an FIR was lodged against the girl's and boy's parents. This order was issued because these functions were superspreaders and they needed to be curbed.'

Chahal adds: 'If the community leader concept had not been created, if he had not been given key functions, if the system had not been coordinated with the 24 war room dashboards, matters would have been worse even in the Delta-led second wave through the 12 months of 2021. We created mechanisms for sanitising washrooms,opening doctor clinics in all the slums areas, facilitating garbage disposal and delivering free grocery and food packets people's to doorsteps. All these put together with thousands of health workers going door-to-door, home-to-home, quarantining high-risk contacts, isolating asymptomatic cases from their existing environment, activating a hospital within Dharavi itself so that patients didn't have to be far from their homes—all this helped a great deal in controlling the spread of the virus among Mumbai's several million slum dwellers. In fact, the International Labour Organization (ILO) lauded Dharavi for its food distribution. We had devised an app, MILKAR, for the distribution of food packets. The ILO picked the MCGM for an award for this innovation.'

A spate of awards greeted Chahal to mark Mumbai's success in combating the pandemic. They included the CNBC-CNN News 18 India Business Leaders Awards (given to Team Dharavi led by Chahal) and the Indo-American Chamber of Commerce (IACC) Covid Crusaders Award. Other awards continued to pour in. The Rotary Club of Bombay wrote[12] to Chahal: 'The board of directors of the Rotary Club of Bombay, a premier Rotary club in India with 92 years of existence, has unanimously approved your name suggested by our Public Awards Committee, as recipient of the Citizen of Mumbai Award for the Rotary year 2020-21.' In the past, the club said, eminent recipients of this prestigious award included former RBI governor Raghuram Rajan and HDFC chairman Deepak Parekh.

The Bombay High Court added its own paean of praise on 6 May 2021: 'The Mumbai Model (as pointed out by the Supreme Court) should also be regarded as a model for other municipal bodies in the state,' stated Chief Justice Dipankar Datta and Justice Girish Kulkarni while deciding a PIL before the bench. As the shortage of oxygen struck Delhi in 2021, the courts again found merit in Mumbai's Covid-19 strategy. *Live Law*, a leading legal website, reported[13] that the Supreme Court had suggested the adoption of the Mumbai Model for Delhi to manage the issue of liquid medical oxygen supply for Covid-19 patients. The Supreme Court observed that the MCGM did well to manage the oxygen situation, and asked if the model could be replicated in Delhi. 'Draw from the experience of the Municipal Corporation of Greater Mumbai; they are doing some great work,' noted a bench comprising Justices D.Y. Chandrachud and M.R. Shah.

Live Law added further context: 'The bench was hearing a petition filed by the central government against the show-cause notice issued by the Delhi High Court for contempt action for failing to supply 700

[12]13 January 2021.
[13]6 May 2021.

MT of oxygen per day to the National Capital Territory of Delhi in terms of the court's" orders. During the hearing, the bench of Justices D.Y. Chandrachud and M.R. Shah suggested the model adopted by Mumbai's municipal corporation be emulated to tackle the issue of oxygen shortage in Delhi. Remarked Justice Chandrachud: "There is a wealth of information coming in every day. Mumbai's municipal corporation is doing some great work, with no disrespect to Delhi. What they are doing, how they are managing. We can learn from them. I also understand that Maharashtra also produces oxygen which Delhi cannot do."

'Solicitor-General Tushar Mehta agreed with the judge and stated, "I do applaud the Mumbai Model. It is not a political model. As an officer of the court, not for centre or state, we need to find a solution. People cannot run from pillar to post. This is not to undermine the efforts of Delhi." The SC continued (in its observations) that the cases in Mumbai were also receding, and that despite similar caseloads, the oxygen consumption in Mumbai was lesser. Mumbai managed with 275 MT of oxygen even when the active cases had crossed 92,000. The SC said that Mumbai was requested to send a model so that other states could emulate the same.'

According to *Live Law,* 'Justice Chandrachud also noted that buffer stocks of oxygen had to be created for emergency purposes. He further suggested that the chief secretaries and health secretaries of both the Delhi government and the central government should have a discussion with the Commissioner of the mumbai municipal corporation to draw from Mumbai's experiences. Justice Chandrachud observed: "If this can be done in Mumbai, which is an incredibly congested city, then it can be done in Delhi as well. If both the chief secretary and health secretary of Delhi and the Centre could converse with the MCGM commissioner and the additional commissioner, if you can draw from that experience, how you can create storage tanks, and buffer storage, etc, if you can do that between today and Monday, we will get a plan in place for Delhi on the Mumbai model, we will have a fairly successful model in Delhi. We want to analyse what was done in a large metropolis like Mumbai and how it can be emulated, as we are answerable to the citizens of Delhi".'

Other courts were equally impressed. Passing an order on 2 May 2021 in a *suo motu* PIL, the Nagpur bench of the Bombay High Court, comprising Justice Sunil Shukre and Justice Avinash Gharote, while dealing with other matters in its judgement, noted pointedly: '(The) authorities may adopt the model devised by the Mumbai municipal corporation under the leadership of its commissioner Mr Iqbal Singh Chahal. For issuance of this order, assistance may be sought from the legal experts including the learned government pleader. Once such a common order is issued, we make it clear that it would be mandatory for all hospitals, whether government, zilla parishad or private or society or trust hospital, to abide by the same and any reluctance or disobedience shown in respect of this order shall be viewed seriously by this Court.'

As the monsoon lashed Mumbai in the first week of July 2020, the city hunkered down. Nature would soon unleash unprecedented fury on the city. It would further complicate the city's battle against Covid-19.

FIVE

THE FORCE OF NATURE

As the first wave of the pandemic peaked, Mumbai was hit by an unprecedented succession of cyclones, storms and flooding. On 23 September 2020, Mumbai received 256 mm rainfall—a record for a single day. August 2020 was the wettest month in over half-a-century. At 3,666 mm of rain, 2020 turned out to be the year with the fiercest monsoon season in the history of Mumbai since 1958 when the city received 3,760 mm of rain in May. The cocktail of Covid-19 and a season of cyclones and storms made 2020 a year of exceptional stress for Mumbai.

Ruminates Chahal: 'I was busy setting up 24 ward war rooms in June 2020, building 8 Jumbo field hospitals, finalising Covid testing regimes, arranging ambulance deployment, getting private hospitals on board, creating a real-time dashboard for the allotment of beds, setting up systems for Covid patients as well as those who were on permanent dialysis, and making sure that quarantine protocols were followed. Our chase the virus policy had met with great initial success. We were moving symptomatic people from containment zones into hotels for quarantining to break the virus chain. It was a challenging exercise which involved the deployment of thousands of health workers.'

With all this frenetic activity, says Chahal, 'There was no time to even imagine that a series of natural calamities were about to hit us hard. The cyclone threat came on 3 June, less than a month after I became the commissioner. On 1 June, I received a message from the regional director of the Indian Meteorological Department (IMD). He said that cyclone Nisarga is active in the Arabian Sea and heading towards Mumbai. It did not register on me at the time that this could be calamitous. I was immersed in fighting Covid. On 1 June, I had spent half a day in the Bombay high court, interacting with the Chief Justice and a number of judges of the High Court, the advocate-general, additional solicitor-general, and others. My presentation lasted for 3 hours. The moment I came out of the high court, I received an SMS from then additional chief secretary Sitaram Kunte. He had been commissioner of the MCGM from 2013-2016. He wrote: "Iqbal, please update yourself on the points decided in the meeting yesterday regarding cyclone Nisarga and take all necessary actions. Mission is zero casualties as stated by the cabinet secretary of India."

'The cabinet secretary held a virtual conference on the impending cyclone on 1 June. Kunte also mentioned something very important to me the next day, 2 June. He said, "Iqbal, as per IMD, cyclone Nisarga will bring additional storms along with tides that will be 2 metres above the normal astronomical tide." That meant an astronomical tide of 4 metres and a storm surge of 2 metres. Thus the total tidal wave could be 6 metres—nearly 20 feet. Kunte said that in his several years in the MCGM, he had not seen such tidal waves. "Please prepare meticulously as this is a very serious situation," he warned.

'When I read Sitaram Kunte's messages on 2 June, I realised the seriousness of the situation. If you have 20-feet-high tides, then it can sweep away the slums of Mumbai which are spread around the sea. That day we decided to have a long 4-hour Zoom conference with all our ward officers, joint commissioners, deputy commissioners, additional commissioners and ward-level staff. Aaditya Thackeray, the guardian minister, decided to join the conference. We had not seen a major cyclone in Mumbai since 1891. Cyclone Nisarga was about to hit Mumbai,therefore, after a gap of 129 years. I decided to ring up my IAS colleagues and batchmates in Odisha, a state which faces cyclones every year. I wanted to learn from their experience. In our control room, we have a disaster management division which is on permanent standby for earthquakes, volcanoes, floods, major fires, tsunamis and other natural calamities. The SOPs are clearly spelt out. But many times people use ingenious methods to confront natural calamities.

'My IAS batchmates in Odisha briefed me on the precautionary steps they take before an impending cyclone. They place tree-cutters in every ward so that collapsed trees can be removed easily to allow access to ambulances and other emergency vehicles. They use gas-cutters and JCB machines to take care of fallen poles. After collating all this information, we started preparing things at the ward level. I told every one of our ward officers that all of us, from the municipal commissioner to the MCGM workers, would be out on the streets when the cyclone, struck Mumbai. Even if we are blown away by the cyclone we have to be on the streets. If I don't see them on the road, I warned, they will be answerable to me. I will be on the road from 8.00 am to 12 midnight.

'That night, Sitaram Kunte, marshalling all the experience he had garnered as the city's municipal commissioner, sent me a message. He said that the wind speed is estimated to be 100 kilometres per hour. Some of our Jumbo medical centres had become operational on 25 May. We had 156 patients in the BKC Jumbo care centre on oxygen on 2 June. The structural engineer had certified the structure for a maximum wind speed of 85 kilometres per hour. The Jumbo would be blown away in the cyclone and 156 Covid patients on oxygen could all die.

'When the MMRDA constructed the BKC Jumbo field hospital, the structural consultants certified that the structure could withstand wind speeds only up to 85 kilometres per hour. So clearly, we were far short of the 100 kilometres per hour wind speed. When we built the field hospitals we had not been fully prepared for a major cyclone. There was no way that in a few hours we could change the Jumbo's structural stability. We then took a bold decision. That night and before the next morning when the cyclone was to strike the city, we deployed a fleet of ambulances. Patients at the field hospitals, including those on ventilators or oxygen, were all shifted to the Worli Dome Jumbo. The Dome is a permanent, reinforced structure. That night, we shifted 156 Covid-positive patients from the BKC Jumbo to the Worli Dome Jumbo hospital. The operation went on through the whole night. Along with the patients, paramedical staff and doctors were also shifted. Put together, around 500 people were moved overnight.'

As cyclone Nisarga threatened the city, the authorities issued an internal memo setting out clear instructions on tackling the impending crisis:

1. Zero casualties should be the target.
2. All hospitals to check backup power supply. Check uninterrupted power supply even if the power lines fail. Check the power generators.
3. Send SMS blasts giving advisory to all people.
4. Shift low-lying area people who are at risk.
5. When the cyclone crosses tin roofs, roof covers might fly off. Slums and temporary structure areas have to be adequately protected.
6. All temporary structures (Jumbo facilities) need to check structural stability considering the possibility of 105 kilometres per hour winds.

On the fraught evening of 2 June, Chahal was constantly in touch with the IMD's regional director, seeking information on the speed, trajectory and direction of the cyclone. 'At 10.30 pm, the regional director called; he told me the cyclone is 50 kilometres away from Mumbai and moving at a speed of 5 kilometres per hour,' Chahal recalls. 'It will take 10 hours to reach Mumbai—by 9.30 am the next morning, he said. I asked the IMD director about the likelihood of the cyclone swerving away from Mumbai. He said the likelihood was zero per cent. I asked him why the cyclone was moving so slowly. He told me that a cyclone sucks in air. Right now it is sucking in air and its speed is slow but then it will explode. I asked him where the cyclone will hit. He said it will make landfall in the northern Mumbai suburb of Andheri. I recalled that over the last 10 days a cyclone had hit Kolkata and there was no electricity in several areas of the city for several days. I was worried: on 2 June, we had 22,000 Covid patients in various hospitals. If the cyclone hit Mumbai dead centre and electricity was disrupted for several days, for how long could our back-up generators work? I knew if a major power outage happened, the lives of many Covid patients would be in jeopardy.

'At 11 o'clock that night, 2 June, Chief Minister Uddhav Thackeray phoned me. He was worried about the impact of the cyclone in the middle of a Covid pandemic. I assured him that along with my ward officers we have decided to fight this crisis come what may. We would not give up the fight. That whole night I couldn't sleep.'

Chahal's IAS batchmates in Odisha, meanwhile, gave him two important pieces of advice. First, they said, when the cyclone hits Mumbai at an estimated wind speed of over 100 kilometres per hour—normally, cyclonic winds start at around 80 kilometres per hour and can go up to 120 kilometres per hour—ensure that major hoardings and trees don't fall and choke major road arteries in the city. When major arteries are blocked by fallen trees and large hoardings, free movement of ambulances, fire brigades and rescue vehicles is affected.

Second, the Odisha-based IAS officers told Chahal to make sure that every ward office and police station kept tree-cutting and metal-cutting equipment ready. Mumbai has scores of police stations and 24 wards. Each should have rescue teams ready. All the equipment plus trained manpower must be deployed before the onset of the cyclone. This would greatly help rescue teams and protect major transport arteries. Mumbai has two major arteries—western and central. If these two arteries are kept free from felled trees and other impediments, ambulances and rescue teams can reach troubled spots quickly.

Chahal was in agreement. 'A cyclone obviously brings heavy rainfall and suddenly you could have a cloudburst,' he says. 'In the monsoon, Mumbai has 380 spots where additional waterlogging takes place because of the structure of that area. The only solution is that when water rises to around 1 foot, our dewatering pumps start throwing water into the nullahs. There are 380 points with dewatering pumps placed permanently in Mumbai. During the last monsoon, we pumped out four times the volume of water contained in Tulsi lake. These are heavy-duty pumps. They have to be stationed in place before the onset of a cyclone with adequate supplies of diesel and a group of engineers monitoring and fixing any breakdowns.

'On 3 June, from 8.00 am to 6.00 pm, I was continuously on the road. We already had with us maps of low-lying areas where landslides could take place, endangering lives during a cyclone and the downpour that follows. We had information on vulnerable slums in low-lying areas where water starts collecting as soon as heavy rain falls. We were already dealing with Covid-19. If 20-feet-high tides hit the slums, they would be swept away. We therefore began a major rescue operation of shifting these vulnerable people in the middle of a pandemic. Our 24 ward war rooms and most of the Jumbo field hospitals were still not operational. Construction of the field hospitals was in full swing and we had to protect them from the cyclone.

'On the night of 2 June, we shifted 48,000 vulnerable people living in slums or shanties in low-lying, flood-prone areas from their homes to nearby municipal schools, mangal karyalayas, marriage halls and dharamshalas. This was a mammoth pre-emptive operation. Moreover, the 48,000 people would have to be housed for 3 days till the effects of the cyclone wore off. They had to be provided breakfast, lunch and dinner. So 48,000 meals were made available 3 times a day with the help of NGOs. All this was taking place on 2 June. The 24 war rooms were to start on 8 June. At that time we had no dashboard, we were just running around the city alloting hospital beds to Covid patients.'

Turning adversity into opportunity, Chahal spoke to the chief minister. Once these 48,000 vulnerable people were under the MCGM's protection, and once the cyclone had passed, Thackeray suggested that they could be tested for Covid en masse. If comorbid conditions were present, they could be treated. It would be a massive health exercise.

Says Chahal: 'I instructed our teams that all comorbid patients under our protection should be sent for immediate testing after the cyclone. If we segregate these most vulnerable people at this early stage, it would give us a great advantage in our fight against Covid-19. We identified several hundred people who were comorbid or had a temperature. Under normal circumstances, we would not have been able to do early Covid testing on this large a scale in a matter of 3 days. The cyclone gave us that opportunity. We also rescued more people from flood-prone areas, began planning for their meals, their relocation, and so forth. The railways were also on board. We gave them SOPs. The railways were told to function as normally as possible in cyclonic conditions.

'That day we spoke to all the deans of private hospitals on video conference. I shared with them what I had learnt from Odisha. We told the private hospital deans that they must be equipped with generator backups since they had patients in ICUs. If there is no electricity, all their machines, including ventilators, would be impacted. We could not afford even a 30-minute breakdown of power. Hospitals and Jumbos were instructed to store 7 days' supply of diesel. Our engineering team was taking care of 147 hospitals, including small ones, equipping them with backups. We were ensuring that they did not run short of diesel or manpower. On 2 June there were 1,500 patients in ICUs and a total of over 20,000 Covid patients in hospitals.

'After I finished speaking to the IMD regional director that night, the chief minister phoned me. He asked me about the preparations we had made. I briefed him on the various steps we had taken to mitigate the risk while tackling both Covid and the cyclone. Finally, the CM asked me one question: "Chahal, what do you think will happen?" I told him that we will do our best but the rest is in the hands of God. I have instructed my team to be on the road at 8.00 am the next day, 3 June.

'It was one of the most difficult nights in my life. We issued a lot of social media messages that night, requesting people not to believe rumours, not to drive any vehicle in the cyclone, to stay indoors, stay away from damaged buildings, not move injured people unless it was absolutely safe to do so, not allow oil and other inflammable substances to spill. Our control room has a screen wall. We have 5,000 cameras all over the city. So each surveilled spot comes up on the full screen. We have 50-plus people constantly monitoring the control room. We told them to inform us immediately if the cyclone causes damage somewhere. In fact, most of us did not sleep that night. I must say the entire MCGM team did a tremendous job.

'For the first time that morning in many, many years, I saw the wind blowing from land to sea, not the other way around. I told the IMD director about this unusual phenomenon. He said the cyclone is sucking in all the air. He warned that we have to be careful for the next 2 hours. Finally, the cyclone made landfall, swerving at the last moment away from Mumbai. The city was saved literally by a hair's breadth. That day, I knew someone up there was looking after Mumbai. We were going to succeed in our escalating battle against Covid.'

At 6 o'clock in the morning on 3 June, Chahal called the IMD director. He told Chahal there was some good news: 'The cyclone is 70 kilometres away but it is facing Uran now, across the harbour from Mumbai, and is slowly moving towards Ratnagiri in thinly populated rural Maharashtra. But Mumbai would not be fully spared. Even a glancing blow from a severe cyclone can cause great damage.'

In the end, Mumbai was saved from the full fury of the cyclone by providence. The cyclone veered off course. But it unleashed a heavy downpour and gale-force winds. Says Chahal: 'We had transported 48,000 people from low-lying areas the previous night. They were given shelter in nearby places where we could house them safely. Ultimately, the cyclone hit Raigad district at a wind speed of 120 kilometres per hour, causing massive damage there. In some districts, it took one full month for electricity to be fully restored. Although it rained very heavily in Mumbai from 8.00 am to 5.00 pm, there were zero fatalities in the city.

'Several hundred trees, though, fell during the storm. Our teams worked through the day. Not a single lane or bylane in Mumbai was blocked. All the fallen trees had been cleared by the end of the day. Despite the unprecedented rainfall, we ensured that there was no loss of life. On the night of 3 June, when things had started settling down, and when I was going to bed, I reminded myself that the IMD had said there is zero probability of the cyclone *not* hitting Mumbai. God rescued Mumbai—even the IMD said it was a miracle the way the cyclone changed direction at the last moment and went south. I told myself that this is the first sign that God is helping us. It was a clear signal from mother nature. We were sure, I believed from that moment on, to win the Covid battle. It gave us a lot of heart. We never looked back after that. 5 days later, on 8 June, the 24 war rooms started functioning. Things would soon change for the better.'

A cyclone was not the only natural calamity that visited Mumbai in the middle of the pandemic's first wave. 'Every monsoon we get one major flooding, usually in July,' says Chahal. 'But we thought this time the downpour has already come with cyclone Nisarga in June. What can be worse than this? We felt sure that the worst was over. Then suddenly on 17 July, it started raining very heavily. One building collapsed in Fort, Mumbai's central business district. It was perhaps a warning of what was to follow.'

Nature clearly wasn't done with Mumbai. The city, still fighting the first wave of Covid-19, had ducked a cyclone in June and weathered the July downpours. Now, in the relatively dry month of August, it was struck by record rainfall.

Chahal describes the sequence of events: 'The 3-day deluge began on 5 August. When the torrent was at its peak, I was sitting in my office. At around 2.30 pm, I suddenly heard an unusual and large noise on the rooftop. I told our officer on special duty (OSD) and Joint Commissioner Chandrasekhar Chore that I had never heard such a huge noise before. It sounded like someone was throwing stones on the building's roof. I walked into another chamber. It was flooded with water. And then when I went out of our building I saw hundreds of tiles from the building's rooftop flying away and hitting another building. That was the loud noise I had heard.'

The wind in south Mumbai had whipped up to 100 kilometres per hour by 3 pm. Chahal drove across the city. Nariman Point was completely flooded. 'Each and every road was like a river,' he says. 'Water was 5-6 feet deep. This was almost like another cyclone—but one which had come without any warning. 'By 5.15 pm, there was knee-deep water in the MCGM's heritage building's main porch. Cars were submerged. The fire brigade arrived. The fire officers said my official car will not be able to reach my home with the roads totally flooded. Entire roads were like rivers. At one place I could see dozens of vehicles submerged. The road had completely disappeared. There were fallen trees all over. Over a thousand trees fell in south Mumbai, the highest ever in Mumbai.'

Chahal says that in such natural calamities, fatalities are usually common. 'Sharad Pawar, whom I have always admired as a brilliant and towering politician, said that in his lifetime of 80 years he had not seen anything as unprecedented as this. Nariman Point is well planned with proper drains and systems in place, but even then it had 4-5 feet of water that day. Pawar was stuck at the Y.B. Chavan Centre. He could not believe the extent of damage caused. I was driving down Churchgate Road. When I reached Marine Drive, I was aghast to see that the road there had totally disappeared. Sea water was touching the walls of the art deco buildings—there was no differentiating between the footpath area in front of the buildings and the main road. This was something I had never seen before and may never see in my life again. Marine Drive was a single sea. Incredibly, however, by early next morning everything had cleared. It was like a flash flood and a cyclone put together.'

Meanwhile, Jaslok Hospital had to keep its windows open. With hundreds of Covid patients inside, many of the hospital's windows were blown away. The worst calamity of the August downpour was that it lifted up the huge retaining wall at Malabar Hill. 'I was shocked,' says Chahal, 'when I went early morning to the site, just short of the Kemps Corner flyover in south Mumbai. I realised that the road had, incredibly enough, moved up by 7 feet from its existing level. I asked our engineers and they said that the Malabar Hill "mountain" had gone down under the road and pushed it up by 7 feet. The retaining wall of the famous Hanging Gardens on Malabar Hill had literally disappeared.'

In the a fortnight following the unprecedented downpour, Tulsi, Vihar and Powai lake levels rose by 140 per cent. The silver lining was that the record rainfall ended Mumbai's water problems which had led to sharp cuts in daily supplies of municipal water. The city received 294 mm rainfall in 24 hours on 5 August. Some areas got 360 mm, breaking a 46-year-old record. It was the wettest August in 62 years.

August was also among the worst months in terms of the numbers of Covid-positive cases in Mumbai. The pandemic continued to rage amidst the most ferocious monsoon in decades. Heavy sanitisation in the slums was increasingly becoming a priority as flooding added to the anxiety caused by rising Covid cases in congested living spaces. 'Fortunately, no other disease was reported by the MCGM during the monsoon season,' says Chahal. 'That was a collateral benefit of the steps we had already taken to sanitise vulnerable areas, especially the slums. All other diseases, except for Covid, had reduced significantly due to overall sanitisation.'

After the August floods, the city thought the worst was over. But on 23 September it started raining heavily again. There was several feet of water on the roads. By 23 September Mithi River was again in spate, causing flooding. From the control room the civic authorities could see all the flooding spots in Mumbai in real-time. In all, there were four major unprecedented floods in Mumbai in 2020: 3 June, 17 July, 5 August and 23 September. Each was a natural calamity, making Mumbai's battle against Covid-19 much more difficult. But in all four calamities there were zero deaths in Mumbai.

'There were a number of takeaways from this experience,' says Chahal thoughtfully. 'First, zero deaths; second, zero impact on our Covid patients and hospitals; third, no fatality of any Covid patient, even indirectly. One of the reasons media criticism of our Covid battle has been muted is the manner in which we handled the natural calamities that struck Mumbai at around the same time as the pandemic's first wave, when the city's health infrastructure was severely stretched.'

It was clear, though, that in order to overhaul Mumbai's civic management, Chahal's MCGM budget speech in February 2021 would need to address the pressing issues. The 2021-22 MCGM budget accordingly allocated 12 per cent of the total outlay to healthcare (₹4,728 crore). That figure would obviously have to increase in the current fiscal year as the civic body races to vaccinate 15 million citizens, including children, before future waves of the pandemic buffet Mumbai.

The key element in Chahal's budget speech was the one most debated: whether Mumbai should have a single planning authority like London or New York. The *Hindustan Times* placed this issue in sharp perspective:

> 'Making the civic body the single planning authority for Mumbai—a proposal sent by the MCGM to the Maharashtra government—could impact redevelopment of buildings, vertical and infrastructure development, while bringing in considerable revenue to the civic body, according to urban planning experts. If approved by the state, it could change the face of development in parts of Mumbai, such as Andheri (East), Goregaon and parts of the east coast, Chembur and Charkop, among others.
>
> 'Currently, the city has multiple planning authorities such as the Mumbai Metropolitan Region Development Authority (MMRDA), the Maharashtra Housing and Area Development Authority (MHADA), the Maharashtra Industrial Development Corporation (MIDC), the Slum Rehabilitation Authority (SRA) and the Mumbai Port Trust (MPT). There are many pockets in Mumbai where the MCGM is not the planning authority. For example, the MMRDA is the planning authority for parts of Bandra Reclamation, Bandra-Kurla Complex and Nariman Point; many areas along the east coast of Mumbai are with the Mumbai Port Trust, the Andheri East area is in the possession

> of MIDC and SRA is the planning authority for all slums in the city from Dahisar to Colaba.
>
> 'These authorities have to be approached for construction permits in these areas. Moreover, premiums and construction charges are paid to these authorities at the time of new constructions or redevelopment. The MCGM's Development Control and Promotion Regulations 2034 do not apply to these areas. Effectively, the Floor Space Index (FSI) that these buildings can avail of differs, and the mandatory open space requirement of a plot, at the time of construction, also differs. However, the MCGM provides all the civic amenities such as water supply, sewerage lines, roads, and no-objection fire certificates to the buildings in these areas.'

Chahal himself is hopeful that reform is possible to make Mumbai a truly global city with coordinated planning by a single authority as he forcefully proposed in his budget speech. Designating the MCGM as the single planning authority, he believes, is imperative.

As Covid-19 continued to wreak havoc, patients with comorbidities were especially vulnerable. Patients on dialysis presented an acute problem. Several of those who were on permanent dialysis for years had tested Covid-positive. Rues Chahal: 'It was a double whammy. On the one hand, they had to have dialysis twice a week and on the other, they had to take a lot of medication. They were highly comorbid. They had no functioning kidneys and were very vulnerable. Many deaths occurred because patients on permanent dialysis suddenly became Covid-positive. Many were admitted into hospitals which did not have dialysis facilities. We had limited beds initially. We started with just 3,000 beds for 15 million people under our jurisdiction in Mumbai. No one was prepared for this once-in-a-century pandemic.

'Our main challenge was to find a bed for everybody. With 15 million people and 3,000 hospital beds, the situation was obviously dire. When a patient is on permanent dialysis with no functioning kidneys and is infected with the coronavirus, the death rate shoots up. If the hospital doesn't have a dialysis facility, the doctors can't move the patient to another hospital with dialysis equipment because he could spread the virus there. Several patients died because of this confusion. In Mumbai, 10,000 people are on permanent dialysis. They suddenly became very vulnerable now.

'I discussed this issue with our medical team and the health department. Around 15-20 people out of 10,000 patients on permanent dialysis were becoming Covid-positive every day. They were very soft targets for the coronavirus. Something had to be done. I was told that 70 nephrologists in Mumbai own dialysis machines which are installed by various doctors in different hospitals. They share the revenue. The key lay with Dr Shrirang Bichu, a world renowned nephrologist and chairman, Apex Kidney Foundation, who coordinated the entire dialysis ecosystem in the city, comprising both equipment and nephrologists.

'As a special case during a public health emergency, Dr Bichu agreed to lower his charges per dialysis patient. I impressed upon him the need to act in the larger national interest. After my fervent appeal guaranteeing him full logistical support, Dr Bichu said he would help us. First of all, he advised, we had to give him a list of hospitals. At that time we had 147 hospitals. He said that he had his own group of nephrologists and would redeploy their dialysis machines to our hospitals. As municipal commissioner, I had to speak to the deans of various hospitals to cooperate with Dr Bichu. If he deployed new machines in their hospitals,the doctors there must assist and support him. There should be no ego clashes. Instead, they should create more space for him. They should create suitable infrastructure for him so that he can install his dialysis machines. Those issues were streamlined.'

As Dr Bichu points out: 'Kidney failure patients require dialysis 3 times a week. If they miss even one dialysis, it can be life-threatening. In late April and early May 2021, several dialysis patients missed their dialysis sessions. Many died, some dialysis centres stopped functioning for various reasons. A large number of patients in dialysis centres started becoming Covid-positive. There was a fear that they may make infect other patients. Dialysis technicians refused to come to work because of the fear of getting infected. Material needed for dialysis was also in short supply. Hence, a large number of patients were left without dialysis. Those dialysis patients who became Covid-positive did not know which dialysis centre to go to. Even if they went to a dialysis centre, they were not receiving slots for dialysis. Municipal Commissioner Chahal supported us in a big way because without the machinery of the MCGM, it would not have been possible at all. It was his idea to create the dialysis portal. *Covidialysis.in* was launched on 20 May 2020 in a record time of just a week under Project Victory.'

Technicians were placed in all the designated hospitals. Dr Bichu held a 3-day training session before they could be redeployed. Chahal gave Dr Bichu a list of 150 technicians. They attended his training programme on how to handle Covid patients on dialysis. Once they were trained, the technicians were deployed in each Covid hospital. It was ensured that every Covid hospital had a dialysis machine. A patient is isolated and cannot move from one hospital to another for dialysis. Once this system was created, Chahal's team came up with a novel idea to save dialysis patients from recurring costs.

'We have a government insurance plan called the Mahatma Jyotiba Phule Insurance Scheme,' explains Chahal. 'If you declare any hospital as being empanelled under this scheme, the hospital starts getting a subsidy of ₹1,500 automatically for every dialysis done there. It was just a piece of paper that needed to be filled up and an order passed that you have been empanelled, irrespective of whether you are a government or a private hospital. All Jumbos were also made to fill up this form. We coordinated with the state health ministry which has the authority to declare hospitals as being empanelled under the Mahatma Jyotiba Phule Insurance Scheme. We placed all the hospitals under this health scheme. The MCGM in the end, had to pay virtually nothing for the dialysis treatment.'

Dr Bichu had, meanwhile, asked for young IIT engineers to design and create the online portal *covidialysis.in*, that Chahal had suggested. The responsibility for monitoring the portal was given to the 70-plus nephrologists who acted as family doctors to the 10,000 Covid patients on dialysis. They had total access to the Covid dialysis portal.

'Dr Bichu has a group of dedicated nephrologists in Mumbai,' notes Chahal. 'These 70 nephrologists have their own subset of doctors. This portal was so well designed by the IIT engineers that we believe it could be among the best anywhere in the world. Now what happens is this: once a person on permanent dialysis is declared Covid-positive through a test and he is symptomatic, he is moved to one of the designated 147 hospitals. He is treated on the first available dialysis machine. When a Covid patient wants his dialysis done at any one of these 147 hospitals, he simply has to make a phone call to his family doctor and tell him that he has been detected Covid-positive and has been brought to this hospital just hours ago.

'The doctor would open the portal, *covidialysis.in*. He would immediately come to know that a certain number of dialysis machines have been installed in specific hospitals. Each dialysis machine has slots for the day. The moment his family doctor books his slot, the patient gets an SMS giving him full details about the dialysis machine and the time slot for his dialysis. Next, the dialysis technician approaches the next patient at the appointed day and time, say 11.00 am, takes the patient to the booked dialysis machine, completes his dialysis and sends him back to his Covid hospital bed.'

There was a complication though. Non-Covid dialysis patients visiting hospitals for their routine dialysis treatment were often shunned. The fear was that they could be asymptomatic for Covid but still infectious. Chahal raised this issue in initial discussions. 'We came up with a solution,' he says. 'We created 2 special hospitals, one in Chembur and another in Ghatkopar, both Mumbai suburbs, for the category of asymptomatic suspected Covid patients who had tested Covid-negative but could be potential carriers. Their doctor could now book their slot in the Chembur or Ghatkopar hospital. We had decided that all asymptomatic non-Covid dialysis patients coming to these hospitals would be regarded as suspected Covid-positive patients and every health worker there would be in full PPE kit. Each time the dialysis was done, the machine was sanitised. And there was a gap of half an hour for the sanitisation to take effect before the next patient was taken in. The Chembur and Ghatkorpar hospitals are like OPDs. They work from 9 am to 6 pm. One machine can do 5-7 dialysis in a day.

'In those days we had to work very fast, there was no question of delays. Till today, several thousand people have benefitted from the *covidialysis* portal. I can safely say that there have been zero deaths due to non-dialysis during the Covid-19 pandemic. We are still continuing with the system. In fact it has become so popular now that it is part and parcel of a dialysis patient's treatment protocol. The portal idea was proposed during discussions with Dr Bichu and the credit goes to the young IIT engineers who created the web portal. This portal is functioning today and helping each and every one of the 10,000 patients in Mumbai who need dialysis—especially those who are also Covid-positive.'

Settling back into his sofa in the spacious commissioner's office, Chahal adds: 'Our unique Covid-19 management system—which, to the best of my knowledge, has not been tried anywhere else in the country—needs an enabling environment which is very difficult to create. We had to come up with unique ideas when the first wave of Covid-19 was at its peak in Mumbai. The 24 war rooms were about to become operational. The constant worry was that although the war rooms started on 8 June and although we today have one of the best dashboards for bed allotment to Covid patients, unless there is continuous vigilance, the system will one day collapse. All government programmes start with great fanfare and then they eventually disappear. We were determined not to let that happen and focused on creating foolproof systems that could work on autopilot. It is easy to create a system, but very difficult to maintain it.'

Maharashtra has around 360 IAS officers. Many are posted across the state as collectors and commissioners. Over 100 officers are posted in Mumbai. Most operate out of Mantralaya, including 55 at secretary-level. 'Of these 100-odd IAS officers,' says Chahal, 'around 10 were coming to work at Mantralaya every day. The rest were sitting at home during the first lockdown. I thought we could deploy some IAS officers as troubleshooters in hospitals which were under pressure. In the end, it was a management model: deploying young IAS officers to monitor hospitals, the dashboard system and other protocols. We had set up these systems with careful planning but they needed to be supervised for efficiency. I was immediately given five IAS officers by then state chief secretary Ajoy Mehta, all young, in the age group of 30-35 years, who had spent 8-10 years in the service and were due to become collectors. Ajoy Mehta has been a great pillar of strength and support for me always. I issued written orders for these five IAS officers, outlining their duties and functions. One officer was put in charge of Nair Hospital, another of Sion Hospital, a third of KEM Hospital, the fourth of the cluster of JJ, St. George and GT Hospitals, and the fifth of 13 peripheral hospitals in Mumbai.

'Each of these five IAS officers was asked to create a war room within the hospital he was put in charge of. CCTV cameras were installed. They covered all the Covid beds in the hospital. There was live surveillance in the control room of all the beds through the CCTV cameras, especially at night. We had received many complaints that after 2.00 am all the doctors, nurses and ward boys would either disappear or go to sleep. In case the patient required help in an emergency in the middle of the night, there was no assistance available. But if the nurses, ward boys and sweepers knew that they were being monitored in the control room through the CCTV cameras, it would improve their attendance, post-midnight to early morning.

'The CCTV cameras in both the regular Covid wards and the Covid ICUs were located in such a way that they showed the presence of doctors, nurses and ward attendents working there. In any hospital, you must be able to see all the beds and the hospital staff round the clock, from the control room. The recording should be preserved. If a complaint is received claiming that from midnight to early morning the staff was not present, we can run the CCTV footage and prove or disprove that claim. Transparency was of paramount importance. We could tell the media to check the footage of the CCTV cameras of that particular day and time in that particular hospital.'

Chahal also mandated that beds for Covid-19 patients must be given a unique ID number. 'Even if we have 30,000 Covid beds showing on the dashboard,' he says, 'every bed has a unique number. If a patient is alloted a hospital, the name of the hospital reflects in the SMS sent to the patient along with the bed number and whether it is an ICU bed or oxygen bed. Now once you have a bed number, even the dean cannot stop you from occupying the bed. This was one of the duties of the five designated IAS officers: to allot bed numbers. It also ensured that bed availability in each hospital was updated every half an hour on the dashboard. The IAS officers were each given three data entry operators to update information on beds in the hospital under their charge.

'Each officer also made sure that any bed, discharged or occupied, had to reflect upon updation of the portal. They had full access to the portal. There is an engineering section in every hospital. It runs the gas supply, electricity, etc. We earmarked a room, got it emptied, and converted it into a hospital control war room, away from the dean's room. Nobody in the engineering or other hospital departments was disturbed by this arrangement. In effect, the IAS officer became chief administrator of the hospital.'

The Indian Council of Medical Research had advised that the moment a patient became Covid-negative, he should be discharged on either the seventh, tenth or fourteenth day, depending on his condition. 'But after recovering from Covid, patients become very weak,' observes Chahal. 'Often ministers, private secretaries, ministers' relatives, VIPs and VVIPs request that they be allowed to stay in the hospital for a few more days. They feel better and safer in the hospital. We told our IAS officers in charge of the hospitals to ease them out because a new patient needing care cannot be denied a bed. They ruthlessly implemented the discharge policy of the ICMR. During the first wave and even more so during the second wave in Mumbai, hospital beds were very precious. We updated the dashboard every 30 minutes in order to allow other critical patients to avail of bed facilities. We could not allow ministers' relatives to overstay in a hospital.

'We also declared that action should be taken to maintain cleanliness in the hospitals by staff and other workers. The dean is the boss. But if something breaks down or there's a problem with power outage, it was the IAS officer's responsibility to take care of it and not put pressure on the dean. We ordered that every washroom is to be sanitised five times a day just like we had mandated in the containment zones. If you have a clean environment, you can fight Covid better.'

The other duty assigned to the five IAS officers was to ensure that good quality food was placed in hospital canteens with the help of NGOs. The civic body tied up with NGOs and companies like Parle. The officers' responsibility was to make the hospital canteen clean and functional. The officers reported to Chahal every evening so that every means were deployed to bring the initial wave of infections under control. The MCGM also made sure that false news was corrected immediately. There were unverified reports and viral videos of dead bodies lying alongside patients, oxygen leaks and 2 patients lying on one bed. Each report was investigated quickly and action taken. Fake news was rebutted.

'One day, the Union cabinet secretary rang me from Delhi early in the morning,' recounts Chahal. 'He said that in a hospital in Jogeshwari, 16 people had died because oxygen had leaked. Oxygen supply had been subsequently stopped. I immediately sent B. Radhakrishnan, an IAS officer, to conduct an inquiry. He rushed there and told me, sir there were 125 people in the ward who were on oxygen, how can a select number of only 16 die? I forwarded this report to the cabinet secretary. All this happened in a few hours. The cabinet secretary called me back and said he agreed that if there were 125 people in the ward on oxygen, how can only a select 16 die? It should be all 125 or none. That is how fake news was corrected.'

The protocol for hospitals managed by the IAS officers and municipal auditors was clearly spelled out by an MCGM notification:

1. Charges for patients for 80 per cent private hospital beds should be levied as per government norms mentioned. If any discrepancy is found, it should be brought to the notice of the MCGM control room/municipal commissioner.
2. Hospitals must display the charges of PPE kits, masks, gloves, etc. on the notice board at prominent places in the hospitals.
3. Patients should be discharged as per the discharge policy of the ICMR.
4. Hospitals must update in real-time bed vacancies. Any discrepancy in data on the MCGM dashboard needs to be reported to the MCGM/Municipal commissioner.

5. Hospitals should not deny beds to walk-in patients. Someone who is unwell and is poor should not be turned away.
6. Municipal auditors at the admission counters must ensure that no asymptomatic patient is given a bed. They should be directed to a Covid Care Centre.
7. For grievance redressal, a dedicated email id has been set up under Director IT, MCGM. Complaints are investigated and suitable action against the owner or trustee of the private hospital should be proposed by the MCGM after the municipal commissioner's approval.

Once the first wave of the pandemic ebbed in January 2021, the five IAS officers, having institutionalised the systems, left the administration to the deans and senior doctors. Chahal confirms: 'Our own deans and doctors took over the hospital war rooms. But this system had worked so well that later a thought occurred to me about the problem of private hospitals overcharging. There are 35 major private hospitals. The hospitals were following our diktat of reserving 80 per cent of their beds for Covid patients. But there were a few black sheep. One or 2 private hospitals were charging excessively. Bombay Hospital and Breach Candy Hospital have ethics, they never overcharge. Some others, however, were charging ₹9,000 a day for a ventilator bed, ₹7,000 for an oxygen bed and ₹4,000 for an ordinary bed. 3 hospitals were the main culprits.

'The MCGM has more than 2,000 audits in a year because we spend nearly ₹40,000 crore ever year. I issued orders and deployed two municipal auditors in every hospital. The MCGM auditors were told to sit at the admission and discharge counters. The IAS officers were at that time still monitoring several hospitals and our auditors worked under their guidance. Except 3 or 4 private hospitals, the rest welcomed our move. They agreed to our request that whenever a patient is discharged, his bill will be shared with the municipal auditor who will check it.'

The private hospitals have a sanction to charge, besides ₹4,000 for beds, separately for PPE kits, oxygen, masks, medication, etc. The municipal auditor checks whether procedures are being followed correctly or not. The auditor displays on a big board at every hospital the charges of various incidentals, masks, gloves, PPE kits and Remdesivir. All rates are declared publicly and unless the auditor clears the bill, it is not released. This came as a relief to patients' relatives. Of the MCGM's 200 auditors, 70 auditors were deployed across 35 private hospitals at two auditors per hospital. Slowly but steadily, complaints of overcharging started disappearing.

Says Chahal: 'You will be surprised to know that there are several hundred cases where crores have been refunded to already discharged patients by private hospitals where overcharging has been established.' The young and enthusiastic IAS officers—Ajit Patil, Madan Nagargoje, B. Radhakrishnan, Sunil Khodvekar and Prashant Nanavare—did a remarkable job. I am grateful to them.'

Meanwhile, scientists wrestled to answer the question: What caused the country's lethal second wave? The Delta variant worsened matters, but other variants had triggered the upward curve of infections in February-March 2021. Former ICMR director Dr N.K. Ganguly, in an interview,[14] provided a cogent explanation: 'The major mutational virus found in approximately 76 per cent of India's 10,000+ samples was the B117 UK variant. This strain is 70 per cent more transmissible. It doesn't target older people who are getting vaccinated and/or sitting at home. It targets people above the age of 29 years who are asymptomatic and who step out of home regularly to work. The other worrisome variants were the Brazilian variant and the South African

[14] *Sunday Mid-day*, 4 April 2021.

variants. However, the first-ever double mutant strain was found in California.

'The double mutant strain has also been found in 206 samples in Maharashtra out of a total of 10,000+ sequencing samples. Essentially, this strain is a combination of two variants—E484Q and L452R. The latter is the most worrisome one. These two mutants, found only through deep sequencing, are such that they are not affected in the same manner (as other variants) by antibodies. Lots of mutational viruses don't survive; most of them go away but some mutants end up establishing themselves. The L452R variant targets a particular gene that is found in people living in India. We do not know how well the vaccine(s) works on this variant. These mutational strains are new, which is why it is only after the results of the current stage of vaccine (rollout) come in that will we know the effect it has on this strain.'

In a joint op-ed[15] with Namita Jaggi, Chairperson, Labs and Infection Control, Artemis Hospital, Gurgaon, Dr Ganguly added:

> 'A partially vaccinated population also puts pressure on the virus to mutate and find more susceptible hosts, compounding the problem. There are worrisome reports coming in of people getting infected after 14 days of the second dose of vaccination, albeit with a less serious disease pattern.'

Dr Michael Ryan, director of the WHO's emergencies programme, had warned in March 2021: 'It's unrealistic to think that the pandemic will end by the year-end. The world's singular focus right now should be to keep transmission of Covid-19 as low as possible. If we are smart, we can finish with the hospitalisations and the deaths and the tragedy associated with this pandemic by the end of 2021. If the vaccines begin to impact not only deaths and not only hospitalisations, but have a significant impact on transmission dynamics and transmission risk,

[15]The *Times of India,* 19 April 2021.

then I believe we will accelerate towards controlling this pandemic.'

The well-known pulmonologist Dr Zarir Udwadia identified[16] four reasons for the second wave that enveloped India throughout much of 2021:

1. '*Complacency*: Indians let down their collective guard. Instead of being bombarded with messages exhorting us to be vigilant, we heard self-congratulatory declarations of victory from our leaders, cruelly exposed as mere self-assured hubris. Let's be honest, we seemed to be doing well at the start of the year not because of any great public health strategy, but merely due to "luck" and the virus biding its time. And then the bad just got worse.
2. '*A different variant*: It was apparent to experts that the new strain in circulation was caused by a variant far more infectious than the initial strain. Yet we still had no clear indication of the genotype of the strain(s) in circulation because we have performed gene sequencing on a paltry 0.1 per cent of our cases. The UK, by contrast, scored a convincing victory against the virus, partly because of the funds committed to daily sequencing of the virus across the country.
3. '*A slow vaccine rollout*: India's initial vaccine rollout proceeded at a glacial pace without any sense of urgency (before it picked up). Despite India being the "vaccine superpower of the world" we faced the frightening spectacle of vaccine shortages, with several vaccine centres reporting very limited stock. Crowded vaccine centres with people jostling for their turn before stocks finish were common (in the initial stages)—I'm convinced many people acquired Covid at crowded vaccine centres, coming down with symptoms a few days after their first dose.

[16]The *Times of India*, 23 April 2021.

This results in vaccines getting a bad name when in reality, neutralising antibodies build up 2 weeks after the second dose. Our innate inability to socially distance, not the vaccine, is to blame. Vaccine hesitancy (in the early stages) was also to blame. The unchecked spread of misinformation—"death by WhatsApp"—is also responsible for Indians' wariness about the vaccine.

4. '*Political miscalculation*: Allowing rallies and large election meetings without any checks, permitting crowds of several hundreds of thousands to gather en masse for the Kumbh Mela strike one as inappropriate. Religious sentiments, nepotism and crowd-pleasing sadly trump basic public health principles and common sense in India.'

As the vaccination programme gathered steam, Dr Shashank Joshi, a member of the Maharashtra Covid Task Force, outlined[17] the state's strategy:

> 'The second surge started very subtly from small, less exposed population clusters in some districts from where it has rapidly spread to the rest of India. We need to vaccinate all vulnerable groups which can succumb to Covid-19, independent of age, but we must also follow vaccine discipline. Our vaccine approach is calibrated, but soon it will become more open and inclusive. The current focus is on saving the lives of the most vulnerable. We may need to innovate strategies to vaccinate, like using family doctors or paediatricians' clinics or mobile vans or vaccine camps as well as avoid wastage by including exceptions in a mindful way.
>
> 'Vaccines confer protection from disease but not necessarily infection. So post-vaccine, even after full doses, we need to wear

[17]The *Indian Express*, 10 April 2021.

masks, avoid crowds and poorly ventilated spaces, maintain physical distancing and sanitise. We shouldn't unmask while speaking and try to avoid crowds when eating. We need to use safer masking strategies like doubling up, using mask braces, ensuring that it is tight and well fitting. There has to be zero tolerance for violators of Covid norms, behaviour and protocols, and we need to have a single-minded determination to conquer this nasty virus. We need to clear the virus from our environment using mind and body strategies and build a strong Covid-free India.'

As the Mumbai Model drew global plaudits, Chahal became the toast of the city. The journalist Malavika Sangghvi wrote[18] about the "chase the patient" approach of the Mumbai Model: '"Once the doctors in the war rooms received confirmation of positive patients, they visited them at their homes, checked their markers and found them an appropriate hospital bed for treatment," Chahal said. "The same ambulance then transported them to the hospital, where a universal subsidised rate had been organised." Sangitaa Advani, founder-director of Skill Shakti Institute, is one among the many beneficiaries of this strategy. When members of her household tested positive, they were pleasantly surprised to receive daily calls from MCGM doctors, enquiring about their condition. "What's more," she said, "they were always polite, professional and caring." The efficiency of Chahal's plan had been further tested when one Sunday the oxygen level of Advani's staff member began dropping alarmingly. Recollecting the episode, she describes it as a miracle. "Within 20 minutes, the MCGM had sent a well-equipped Covid ambulance and transported the patient to a Jumbo centre." That wasn't all. Once admitted, the patient was made

[18]*Hindustan Times*, 21 May 2021.

comfortable and received nourishing timely food and medicines. Most importantly, he received humane, thoughtful care from the entire medical team, said Advani. When Chahal was appointed as the head of MCGM, he recalls thinking, "A pandemic like this comes once in a century. Hundred years before me and hundred years after me, no municipal commissioner will get this opportunity to serve humanity and save thousands of lives. Maybe I am the blessed one chosen by God."'

Sangghvi concluded her piece: 'If only Chahal's mother had given birth to another hundred like him.'

Though cases and mortalities in Mumbai fell towards the end of 2021, Chahal remained wary about letting the city's guard down. The hiatus between the first and second waves had led to Covid-negligent behaviour. That played a part in the steep rise in Covid cases in April and May 2021 before subsiding. Naandika Tripathi underlined[19] key points in Mumbai's Covid-19 battle and the need to avoid complacency:

> 'Despite the initial chaos, the Mumbai Model of Covid-19 management worked well in the face of the surging second wave and earned praise from the Supreme Court as well. Planning, delegation and launching the right initiatives, like the 24/7 war rooms equipped with doctors and trained staff, worked well in the favour of the MCGM. But it isn't looking to be complacent, instead it has already started preparing for the third wave by training paediatricians, since children are expected to be more vulnerable to the third wave.'

Because the coronavirus and its variants can pose long-term and unpredictable risks, Nitin Desai suggested[20] that the government should shift its focus from pure economic management to public service management:

---

[19] *Forbes India*, 16 June 2021.

[20] *Business Standard*, 29 June 2021.

'The latest National Family Health Survey shows a significant deterioration in the proportion of stunted children. *The Annual Status of Education Report* continues to show the poor outcomes of schooling. The great divide between the rentiers who have inherited wealth, the owners and managers of corporations, the educated and high-skilled elite workforce and the 80 per cent of the population who constitute the rest is growing. Health, education, poverty, employment and environment surveys should provide the real metric of progress rather than stock market indices and GDP growth.

'When it comes to economic policy, the government should set up a sensible, stable and predictable structure of taxes, tariffs and regulations, and leave the rest to the market. The primary task of the government should be to boost the quality and reliability of public services for health and education, provide credible social protection to low-income households, particularly wage labourers at the lower end of the income spectrum and limit its sectoral interventions in the rest of the economy to countering externalities like environmental deterioration arising from private activities.'

Chahal was quick to recognise the power of the print, digital, electronic and social media to mould the narrative. The challenge Chahal faced right through the first wave of the pandemic was providing relevant information on Covid-19 quickly to as large an audience as possible. A colleague gave him an idea: why not use multiple groups on social media, like the WhatsApp platform to disseminate data on the coronavirus? Chahal embraced the idea and expanded it.

On 15 June 2020, he set up over 30 groups on WhatsApp, each targeting specific audiences: journalists, bureaucrats, politicians, judges, diplomats, legislators, even Bollywood stars. More than

6,500 people were included in these 30 groups. The impact was immediate. The media group, for example, has nearly 300 editors and correspondents across print, television and digital media globally.

Foreign journalists were also part of the media group. When authentic information on the pandemic in Mumbai needed to be obtained rapidly, global newspapers such as the *Washington Post,* the *New York Times* and the *Guardian* as well as TV networks like the BBC and CNN communicated with Chahal in what was effectively a two-way information channel. By attaching the real-time, graphic-loaded dashboard with the latest data on cases, deaths, available hospital beds, oxygen, ventilators and ICUs, Mumbai's reputation for transparency grew.

There were additional links to reports on cyclones, flooding and other civic issues. Chahal would regularly update the cabinet secretary of India, the Union home secretary and the Union health secretary. 'I must mention that all of them have consistently encouraged me with appreciation,' says Chahal.

As a broadcast platform, the 30 WhatsApp groups, with a primary influential audience of 6,500, supplemented by the MCGM's regular print and television campaigns as well as its outreach on multiple social media platforms, continue to provide swift and accurate information on the vaccination rollout and ongoing preparations for subsequent waves of the pandemic.

The major stakeholders in Mumbai—opposition political parties and elected office-bearers of the MCGM—were also regularly updated by Chahal. Most were quick to acknowledge the effort and achievements of Team MCGM. Chahal says the Leader of the Opposition and former chief minister Devendra Fadnavis was very supportive and stood behind him and his team. He also provided critical appraisal through the pandemic, which helped Team MCGM to perform at an optimum level.

Chief Minister Uddhav Thackeray's regular Facebook Live video posts enjoyed a wide audience as well and helped allay disquiet among the people as the pandemic underwent wave after wave of infection, hospitalisation and fatality. The WhatsApp broadcasts also helped to correct fake news or slanted reportage. Retractions were quick.

Several stories in the global media examining and lauding the Mumbai Model originated from information and data broadcast by Chahal to the 30 groups and their global audience. It helped counter much of the negative press the Indian response received internationally to the second wave of the pandemic.

Chahal's accessibility to the media allowed him to clear up several misconceptions about Mumbai's long and difficult battle against Covid-19. Speaking to the senior journalist Barkha Dutt on her online news channel, Mojo, as the second wave erupted, Chahal remarked: 'When I took over as commissioner, the slums of Mumbai, especially Dharavi, were on fire. We were getting 300 cases from Dharavi and 1,500 cases from Mumbai on a daily basis. There were dead bodies on the morning of 8 May, in autorickshaws, on footpaths, on road dividers. So the first 15 days were very harrowing. It was the worst fortnight of my life.'

Asked how he reacted on 16-17 April 2021 when 168 patients in 6 hospitals had to be moved due to an oxygen crisis, Chahal replied: 'That was the toughest night. We had all worked so hard for the past one year, and that single night would have washed everything away. What happened was that at 12.30 am, just after midnight, I received a call that 6 hospitals with 168 patients in 34 ICUs have only 2 hours of oxygen left. If we don't shift them immediately, then they will all die. We swung into action immediately. I salute my team. We immediately moved over 150 ambulances. We had them on the Uber software. We also had 3,600 beds, vacant beds, in our Jumbos, out of which 850 were oxygen beds. That is why we were able to shift them, all 168 patients. Otherwise it would not have been possible. So, between 1.00 am and 5.00 am we shifted these 168 patients in an equal number of ambulances. There were 200 MCGM employees deployed in this exercise. I am happy and satisfied that we could save each and every human soul.

'Even today, the media has not reported a single death from that overnight operation. By 5.00 am, when we had successfully completed the operation, I was still very worried. I had 21,000 Covid patients with me and this situation may arise again tonight and every night. So I rang alarm bells everywhere in Mumbai and Delhi. Unless something is done about oxygen supplies immediately, these problems are going to reccur again and again and things could get out of control. I told all my leaders in Mumbai and Delhi that I could not buy oxygen, issue tenders for oxygen, procure oxygen. I was feeling totally helpless. But I am happy to say that the problem was solved that day itself when we got an allocation from Reliance Industries in Jamnagar. The shortage of oxygen has become history since then.'

Chahal explained to Dutt the strategy he employed during the oxygen crisis: 'I went back to my task force and asked them how to save on oxygen. They gave me four points. One, don't maintain saturation levels beyond 94; two, don't use the guzzlers or a high flow of oxygen unless really required; three, tell hospitals to do a weekly oxygen audit. Do the last week's audit and the present week's audit, see how oxygen can be conserved. We started doing this with all the hospitals and it helped us save 10 per cent on oxygen supplies.

'Now when the oxygen tanker leaves the facility of Jindal or Reliance then the instructions must be crystal clear. There should be no overlapping of instructions as to whose tanker it is. Once it comes to Thane in the MMR area, there should be clarity about allocation, clarity about distribution to hospitals, clarity about emergency stocks of oxygen, and clarity about SOPs. During the first wave, the word oxygen was not even discussed in India, as no one felt the shortage. Even we in Mumbai did not feel the shortage. But learning from this, when a similar Covid tsunami strikes again we'll be ready. In the Jumbos, we have put up oxygen plants so that we become self-sufficient and don't bother the central or state government for oxygen.'

Speaking to Dutt about the MCGM's preparations for paediatric facilities, Chahal reiterated: 'Our expert task force has warned us that the next wave may be a paediatric wave. Just imagine if a 4-year-old child becomes Covid-positive and is symptomatic. The child cannot go alone to the hospital. The mother has to go with the child. This requires privacy. So we have built hundreds of cubicles within the Jumbos where the mother and child can have privacy. The best paediatric doctors of Maharashtra have defined SOPs and protocols for home quarantine for children and for hospitalised children.'

In an interaction with *The Print*'s Shekhar Gupta, again at the peak of the second wave, Chahal pointed out that in the second wave, unlike the first, many among the rich and the super-rich were testing positive: 'These people are very impatient, the moment their swab is taken they put so much pressure on the labs to get the test report.' Chahal added: 'The reason why Mumbai did not dismantle any of its Jumbo facilities is direct proof that we were anticipating another wave. NESCO, Goregaon which has 3,000 beds and 224 ICUs, at one time in January had only 3 patients. The dean came to me saying we have only 3 patients, shall we shut it down? I told him no, it must be kept functional. This was just a month before the second wave struck. Not one bed was closed even though we were getting only 200-300 cases in November, December, and January. So we had anticipated the second wave. We are anticipating a third wave and have built four new Jumbos.'

Despite Chahal's media outreach, tendentious reportage in the foreign media continued. Chahal's "broadcast" strategy helped counter clearly erroneous media stories, especially as India—and Mumbai—turned the corner in the fight against the pandemic. The narrative gradually changed. The foreign media's narrative, however, remained skewed against India.

Commenting on Prime Minister Modi's Independence Day speech on 15 August 2021, which focused on India's Covid-19 challenge, the BBC displayed customary asperity: 'Indian Prime Minister Narendra Modi praised healthcare workers and scientists for helping India fight Covid-19 as the country celebrated the (beginning of the) 75th year of independence. Mr Modi also paid tributes to those who died of the virus, saying, "The pain of losing them will stay with us forever". He added that the country fought the virus "with extraordinary pace".

'But his government faced criticism when India's second Covid wave ravaged many towns and cities in April and May 2021.The second wave left millions of people infected and overwhelmed the country's fragile healthcare system to the point of collapse. People died gasping for breath as hospitals ran out of beds and oxygen—leaving distraught family members pleading for help on social media. Even crematoriums in some cities ran out of space.

'Mr Modi also spoke about his vision for India's development, saying the next 25 years will mark the country's growth story. He talked about boosting manufacturing and exports, encouraging home-grown industries and promoting innovation. For this, the prime minister said, the government would launch an infrastructure plan worth $1.35 trillion (£983 billion). The aim is to ensure that the benefits of the economy should trickle down to every village and town in India, he added.

'But Mr Modi's promises come at a time when the Indian economy is struggling to recover from the damage caused by the coronavirus. Growth had been faltering even before 2020 and the pandemic has made matters worse. India's GDP shrunk by an unprecedented 7.3 per cent in the previous financial year as the pandemic wiped out businesses. The virus has left deep scars—unemployment is on the rise while inflation remains high. The government has repeatedly spoken of achieving a sharp recovery in the coming months. But several financial institutions, including the World Bank and the International Monetary Fund, have revised expectations downwards.

'In recent days, Mr Modi's biggest challenge has been to tackle the growing discontent among India's farmers who are angry with a set of new laws aimed at reshaping the country's agriculture industry. Tens of thousands of farmers have been camping on the outskirts of Delhi since November in protest against these laws.'

On the economy and the farmers' protests, the BBC presented a one-sided picture. The green shoots in the economy found no mention and the fact that the farmers' protests were confined largely to Punjab and Haryana received short shrift. The BBC also failed to note that despite India's complex logistics, it was administering in August 2021 an average of more than 5 million doses of Covid-19 vaccines per day—over five times the number in the United States with its relatively advanced healthcare infrastructure. Between September and December 2021, that number rose to a daily average of over 7 million doses, on target to fully inoculate almost all adult Indians by the first quarter of 2022 as well as a significant section of children below the age of 18.

Most responsible Western media organizations eventually got the successful Mumbai Model narrative right, largely due to the swift and transparent information broadcast by Chahal and his team as well as by credible sections of Indian digital, electronic, print and social media.

SIX

NAILING THE VIRUS

While the global and Indian media lauded the Mumbai Model, few recognised the complex factors that made it succeed in a challenging urban agglomeration. Explains Chahal: 'We developed a unique strategy in Mumbai to tackle Covid-19. It was the only city which adopted this model and continues to do so even as successive waves ebb. This is one of the main reasons why our death rate is low despite the surge in waves throughout 2021. The Mumbai Model relies on tracing, testing and treating at a high level of intensity and volume. The success of the Mumbai Model showcases the stellar performance of Team MCGM, 24/7. Let me rewind a bit. In the second week of May 2020, following the central government's direction that we test only symptomatic patients, we prescribed a proforma for medical prescriptions. That proforma was to be signed by the doctor in charge of the clinic. It involved tracing, testing and treating asymptomatic patients in separate sections, even as the vaccination programme rolled out. This reduced both positivity and death rates well into the end of 2021.

'First the doctor had to certify that a patient's swab has been taken and has been recommended for testing. The testing then takes place. The doctor has to certify that the patient has distinct Covid symptoms like loss of taste, temperature, bad throat, etc. The last sentence in the proforma states that if the clinic's doctor is found to have prescribed any medication, then his licence/registration would be cancelled. The certificate reassured the central government that we had no intention whatsoever of hiding positive cases by suppressing the symptoms of the patient.

'When we started testing symptomatic cases, two things happened. One, in a city like Mumbai, even if you test thousands of people in a population of 15 million under the MCGM, there is a possibility that a large number of people who are unwell will get left out. Two, many asymptomatic people suddenly develop symptoms and become breathless. The virus and its variants are very lethal. If in the morning you develop symptoms, and in the evening you become breathless, you may even die later in the night. It can happen that quickly, especially for comorbid patients. During one of the late-night cabinet meetings, the close aide of one senior minister died suddenly. He had become unwell but could not get tested. He did not get a bed in a hospital and he passed away. The cabinet minister was visibly upset. Our system was not taking care of people who were dying of Covid like this.

'This case happened in mid-June 2020. By them our BKC, NESCO and Worli Dome Jumbos had become operational. They had huge capacities. So we came up with the unique idea of creating a separate section of beds for the *suspected* category of patients—similar to what we had done by demarcating 2 special hospitals for dialysis patients suspected to be asymptomatic Covid carriers. We created 2,000 beds which were marked for only suspected Covid cases. We did aggressive publicity for this through the 24 ward war rooms. We said that any patient whose Covid test had not been conducted or whose swab test report was awaited but who felt unwell or got breathless, should call up the nearest ward war room and ask for an ambulance or simply take an auto or a taxi and come to our Jumbo hospitals. Patients in north Mumbai could walk into NESCO Goregaon. Those in mid-Mumbai could go to BKC. Those in south Mumbai could go to Worli.

Those in the eastern suburbs could go to the Mulund Jumbo centre or the Mahalaxmi centre.'

Deans at these Jumbos were instructed that the moment a patient came in an ambulance or a private vehicle, taxi or auto, no questions should be asked. He must be admitted to the bed reserved for suspected Covid patients. He should immediately be put on oxygen and stabilised whether he is Covid-positive or not. Once he was stabilised, he could be tested. 'Oxygen is like a lifeline,' says Chahal. 'These, therefore, were only oxygenated beds. Once the Covid test was conducted, the result would be positive or negative. If positive, the patient would be moved to the Covid section of the Jumbo. If negative, once he had recovered after 3-4 days, he would be discharged. We created 2,000 beds in Mumbai for the Covid-suspected category. This is how we neutralised the deficiency in testing. On 3 July 2020, we began universal testing. Anybody could get a Covid test done without a prescription. Testing numbers shot up. The labs were also upgraded. New labs came up and capacities increased.'

Across India, the prognosis, however, was mixed. Omkar Goswami, chairman of the Corporate and Economic Research Group (CERG), explained[21] in clear scientific terms why the novel coronavirus has exacted such a high national toll:

> 'Just as babies grow teeth, viruses multiply and mutate. After a virus enters a body, it begins a two-pronged battle. One is against the antibodies that are fighting to snuff it out. The other is to mutate and multiply in the host and create more invaders. The novel coronavirus, Sars-CoV-2, is an RNA virus, with ribonucleic acid as its genetic material. Human diseases

[21]The *Economic Times,* 1 May 2021.

caused by RNA viruses include the common cold, influenza, severe acute respiratory syndrome (SARS), Middle East respiratory syndrome (MERS), Covid-19, dengue, hepatitis C, hepatitis E, West Nile fever, Ebola, rabies, polio, mumps and measles.

'Now comes the big problem. RNA viruses have high mutation rates vis-à-vis the DNA virus. This is because viral RNA polymerases (enzymes that synthesise chains of polymers or nucleic acid) do not proofread like DNA polymerases. So, while there are more "errors" in an RNA virus' replication, its speed of reproduction makes it a formidable enemy. Sometimes, these error-prone mutations effectively extinguish the disease-fostering capability of the virus. Equally, the mutations can make the next version more lethal than before.

'This is why flu shots change every year. Ingredients in new shots adjust to deal with the genetic variations that have occurred in the virus during the year. Sars-CoV-2 first mutated in China from bats to humans. Since then, there have been at least five significant mutations. The first, detected in February 2020, spread to quickly become the dominant strain. The second or the UK variant, Alpha, spread through Britain and accounted for some 30 per cent of all Covid-19 infections in England. The third, or the South African variant, originated in October 2020 with increasing powers of transmission. The fourth was the Brazil variant.

'The fifth variant, Delta, was detected in India in late 2020, and is believed to have been the cause behind our second wave. Called B.1.617, it is a double-mutant variant. From virtually nothing this January, the average prevalence of B.1.617 surged to over 50 per cent in samples sequenced nationally in April 2021, and over 60 per cent in Maharashtra. The two mutants in this variant are believed to not only increase transmission, but also reduce the ability of human antibodies and drugs to neutralise the viral effects.'

Binayak Dasgupta and Anonna Dutt added to Goswami's erudite thesis[22]: 'In March 2020, when the world first caught a glimpse of the devastation that the coronavirus would go on to unleash, experts feared India would suffer heavily as well. Tried-and-tested epidemiological models predicted 97,000-1.3 million infections by mid-May 2020, to perhaps even 300 million infections by the end of the year. But, largely, the worst of the fears did not pan out. During the highest of the infection peaks, hospitals appeared to be on top of the situation—unlike in New York or Milan. The season of festivals, which touches almost every region, religion and custom in the pre-winter months of October-November, led to spikes, but not of the nature seen in other parts of the world. Reported cases mean very little in India. The estimated number of true infections from models as well as sero surveys is huge and point to about 20-25 per cent of the adult population being infected. "That is nearly 170-200 million infections," said Bhramar Mukherjee, the chair of biostatistics at the University of Michigan School of Public Health. Even if one takes this into account and looks at fatalities to calculate what is known as the infection fatality rate (IFR), she added, India's story seems different. "Even if you believe not all deaths were reported, this points to a low IFR compared to the rest of the world," she added.

'India's IFR is 0.1 per cent and this number may be a better measure of an epidemic since deaths are more likely to be recorded than infections, particularly in the case of a disease like Covid-19, which infects many without symptoms. But, Mukherjee added, "41 per cent of India's population is

[22]*Hindustan Times*, 1 March, 2021.

> in the age group 0-18, in which the infection rate is really low—so the age-adjusted mortality does not look as low as the overall one."'

Even before the second wave struck India, senior doctors advised both vigilance and caution. Dr Devi Shetty, founder of the Narayana group of hospitals, is one of India's leading medical practitioners. He cautioned[23]: 'Covid is not going to disappear totally for quite some time. Vaccination against Covid will be a long-term affair. Over 500 million Indians need to receive two doses of the vaccine. People I've spoken to thought vaccinating half a billion people with both doses will not be possible. Those same people would have thought providing health insurance to half a billion people wasn't possible. Our doctors, nurses, technicians and healthcare workers did a phenomenal job saving millions of precious lives. They are tired and want to get back to their normal lives. We simply can't afford to go through another Covid peak and lockdown. If we act fast, we will prove to the world that health doesn't depend on the wealth of the nation.'

Questions about critical oxygen supplies in future waves, however, persisted. In an Idea Exchange session with *The Indian Express*[24], Chahal explained how Mumbai overcame oxygen shortages that paralysed Delhi and other cities during the summer of 2021: 'The issue of oxygen first came up at a meeting around the first week of April 2021. It was said that Maharashtra's total installed oxygen capacity is roughly 1,200 MT, which included oxygen for industrial, non-Covid and Covid use. By 5 April, the state's 6 lakh positive cases had started consuming almost 950 MT of oxygen. In our meeting, it was projected that by 15-20 April, our consumption may go up to

[23]The *Times of India,* 19 February 2021.

[24]6 May 2021.

1,700 MT. That is when the alarm bells went off. We realised that even if we stop all industrial operations as well as non-Covid oxygen use, we would still not be able to manage a capacity beyond 1,200 MT of oxygen. So we requested the government of India to give us an additional allocation of 500 MT. About 150-200 MT of this additional allocation was coming from Haldia in West Bengal. For the tanker to reach Mumbai, the turnaround time was around 8 days.

'In the midst of these discussions, on the intervening night of 16-17 April, I was informed around midnight that 6 hospitals were running out of oxygen. There were 168 patients there. As I've already described, between 1.00 am and 5.00 am, we deployed 150 ambulances and brought these patients to our Jumbo Covid centres. Fortunately, we had 3,600 empty beds, of which 850 were oxygenated beds. I was relieved that no lives were lost. After the operation, I couldn't sleep at all, and at around 7.00 am, I sent messages to some of the top functionaries of the government of India, including the principal secretary to the prime minister, the cabinet secretary, the home secretary and the health secretary. I sent another set of messages to the top eight leaders of Maharashtra, starting with the chief minister. I said to them, this is not the end of the problem and this may happen again.

'Within 15-20 seconds, I had an incoming call coming from the cabinet secretary, Rajiv Gauba. He told me, tell me what you want. I said we have to import oxygen into the state. I told him that we can't manufacture oxygen at such short notice and that the turnaround time for oxygen coming from Haldia was around 8 days. I had worked under Gauba when I was joint secretary in the ministry of home affairs. I told him that Reliance Industries was just 16 hours away from Mumbai, in Jamnagar, and oxygen tankers can come from there every night. He said that such an allocation cannot be made just for one city. I told him that he can allocate it to Maharashtra and I will make sure that it comes only to Mumbai city. And then shortly thereafter,

125 MT of oxygen was allocated to us from Reliance Industries in Jamnagar. The same evening, tankers started moving and the problem (of oxygen) became a problem of the past in Mumbai because of the prompt help we received from the government of India.' Chahal adds thoughtfully: 'I hold Rajiv Gauba in high esteem. He is an extremely dynamic and brilliant officer. His lightening response floored me. I shall remain indebted to him.'

Maharashtra too, met the oxygen crisis head-on. The state was starved of oxygen at the height of the second wave. According to Priyanka Kakodkar[25] 'Maharashtra grappled with an alarming reality:

> '50 metric tonnes of oxygen that it had been receiving from a plant in Bellary was no longer going to be available. Yet, in a few hours, a crisis was averted. By dawn, supplies were arranged from Gujarat's Jamnagar and Dolvi and Murbad in the state. As a result, western Maharashtra, which was seeing a spike in cases, was spared an oxygen shortage.
>
> 'Working behind the scenes was a task force of officials fire-fighting through the day to ensure that the state plugs its oxygen crunch and supplies are transported all over. The state's Oxygen Team includes FDA commissioner Parimal Singh, medical education secretary Saurabh Vijay and transport commissioner Avinash Dhakne. They look after the overall allocation to districts, assess demand and organise inter-state transport.
>
> 'The next rung in the Oxygen Team includes nodal officers, each in charge of two revenue divisions. Ashwin Mudgal, joint managing director of CIDCO, is in charge of Vidarbha's Nagpur and Amravati division. Animal husbandry commissioner Sachindra Pratap Singh oversees Marathwada and western

[25]The *Times of India,* 11 May 2021.

> Maharashtra while Amit Saini, CEO of Maharashtra Maritime Board, is in charge of Konkan, MMR and Nashik. Each official also coordinates the supply from another state. The team reports to Chief Secretary Sitaram Kunte in a nightly review meeting at 10.00 pm. "This is a crucial meeting in which the demand, supply and emergencies are assessed," said a senior officer.'

Despite a heavy caseload, Mumbai did not suffer from a major oxygen crisis during the infectious second wave. The MCGM's Additional Municipal Commissioner P. Velrasu explained[26] why Mumbai's efforts bore fruit:

> 'The MCGM started with resource mapping and inventory accounting from May 2020 itself, following oxygen difficulties in one of our hospitals within months of the Covid outbreak in Mumbai. Our Oxygen Team was asked to visit every hospital and compile data on shortage capacity, supply method, suppliers' name and supply periodicity. We accounted for a much increased oxygen demand during the pandemic and expected the number of ICU and oxygenated beds to go up. The next step was to increase the shortage capacities by installing additional cryogenic tankers in civic hospitals. The work was completed within 40 days. Underutilised during the first Covid-19 wave, the tank took the load during the second Covid-19 wave very effectively.'

Chronic problems, however, continued to beset the city. Following oxygen shortages in several hospitals earlier in the year, Chahal ordered a new protocol:

[26]The *Times of India*, 7 May 2021.

'According to the new system[27], a data sheet with details of all private hospitals, Covid hospitals, their respective suppliers along with data on dura, jumbo and small oxygen cylinders available at the hospitals will be provided to the ward control room and the Food and Drug Administration's (FDA) control room. Hospitals would have to request oxygen from suppliers at least 24 hours in advance or as per their agreement, whichever is earlier. If this supply is not available within 16 hours, the hospital would have to inform the ward office's control room, which will contact the supplier to ensure timely delivery. If the supplier cannot provide it within 2 hours, the ward control room would contact the FDA's control room.

'The FDA control room would then speak to the supplier. If the oxygen still cannot be made available within 2 hours, the FDA would have to contact the coordinating executive engineer of the ward, who'd have to bring oxygen to the hospitals. All medical officers shall inform the Covid hospital in their jurisdiction to ensure smooth supply. Assistant municipal commissioners have to inform medical officers and control room officers of the ward about the procedure. The executive health officer should inform all hospitals. It is also directed that all concerned hospital take due diligence and responsibility to ensure proper supply as per number of patients.'

When warnings about the second wave were sounded in February 2021, few took note. By early February cases in Mumbai had dropped significantly. A second wave seemed improbable. Within weeks the mood darkened as cases began to rise, first in Mumbai and then in

[27] *Mid-day*, 24 April 2021.

other cities. In a prescient analysis, *Hindustan Times* editor-in-chief R. Sukumar wrote[28]:

> 'That there is a second wave of the coronavirus pandemic is now certain. The 7-day average of daily cases on Thursday night was 29,330, 167 per cent higher than its post-first wave peak low; and the 7-day average of daily deaths, 151, 71 per cent higher. Maharashtra, Punjab, Haryana, Madhya Pradesh, Tamil Nadu, and Andhra Pradesh are all seeing a resurgence in cases. And despite Prime Minister Narendra Modi's exhortations and warnings in the course of a video conference meeting with chief ministers on Wednesday, no one really seems to care.
>
> 'The second wave, if left uncontrolled, could surpass the peak of the first wave, as the experience of other countries shows. The fact that it is raging at a time when new variants of the coronavirus disease, including the dangerous P1 variant that is wreaking havoc in Brazil, have all been sequenced in India, is cause for concern. The situation now is far more dire than it was exactly a year ago, when India started thinking about a lockdown, and finally implemented one at 4 hours' notice on 25 March 2020.
>
> 'Given this context, what should India's response be? A nationwide lockdown is out of the question for two reasons—its impact on a still-fledgling economic recovery would be catastrophic; and after a year of living with the SARS-CoV-2 virus, it is clear that other measures can achieve the same result as a hard lockdown. It is time for the Union health ministry and the drug regulator to approve more vaccines. If the latter could approve Bharat Biotech's Covaxin on the basis of belief and not hard evidence—as expected by many, the evidence

[28]20 March 2021.

> followed, and showed the vaccine to be highly effective, but vaccines should always be approved on the basis of science, not belief—there's no reason for it to drag its feet over the Sputnik vaccine, or the Novavax one, which will be made in India by the Serum Institute of India. And once approved, it should allow their sales in the open market.'

Indeed, more vaccines, home-grown and imported, were swiftly approved by Indian regulators as the vaccination drive accelerated between September and December 2021. The second wave cascaded through India, reached a peak in May-June 2021 and ebbed, but haltingly, towards the end of the year. That indicated how important it was to maintain a high degree of vigilance. In Mumbai, scalded by the second wave, caution was the watchword.

Mission Save Lives was a key strategy adopted by the MCGM to keep the city's guard up. Chahal elaborates: 'We had convened a team of doctors to study and tell us why the death rate was initially relatively high in Mumbai. What could be the reasons for high mortality rates? What should we do to counter this? The study conducted by these doctors found that most of the patients were on oxygen. If they wanted to use the washroom late at night, it was quite natural that our ward boys and nurses would not be that vigilant. They even tended to go to sleep. Our CCTV cameras had not yet been installed in all the medical centres.

'The study found that when patients with oxygen masks went to the washroom, they used their own hands to remove the oxygen masks to walk down several metres to the nearest toilet. They used the washroom for 2-3 minutes. By the time they came back, it was another 4-5 minutes. Now during this period, supposing their oxygen level was already low, say 70-75 per cent, the body immediately, in 2-3 minutes, starts reacting to the low levels of oxygen. We received a number of complaints about senior citizens, especially patients in their 70s, being found dead in hospital toilets. There were even cases of patients who would collapse on the hospital floor on their way back to their beds. Such unfortunate deaths happened in KEM, Sion and Nair Hospitals.

'We therefore drafted an order and launched Mission Save Lives. The new strategy covered all aspects necessary to achieve this goal and further strengthen the healthcare system and administration. We also had to ensure that all treatment protocols were followed. There was a mismatch between senior and junior doctors. In government hospitals, we have deans and heads of departments (HODs) as well as young residents who are doing an MD or an MS in a speciality. They are the ones who run the show. If there is a disconnect between them and the deans, there will be problems. So we made it compulsory that deans and HODs must interact with the young resident doctors twice a day over video conferencing. For example, if a young resident doctor is looking after 10 patients in a particular ward, he or she must discuss what kind of medicines are being prescribed to the patients and if any change is required or other intervention needed. The HODs and the deans must interact with them.'

Healthcare experts observed that several deaths were taking place between 1.00 am and 5.00 am. As expected, this was the time period when patients remove their oxygen masks to go to the toilet. Chahal passed an order that every bed should have a commode or a bed pan. The ward boys on duty must assist the patient in using the bedpan. This bedpan should be under each patient's bed and could be used without removing the oxygen mask. 'This saved many lives,' says Chahal. 'I will give one example. This procedure was implemented on 1 July and immediately on 4 July, the columnist Shobhaa De published an article on Mission Save Lives.'

She wrote: 'Amidst all these morbid stories comes a simple, practical suggestion from the municipal commissioner with focus on the Mission Save Lives initiative which concentrates on reducing mortality rates in hospitals. Every bed should have a bedpan and every 4 beds should have a commode. A study shows that a high number of Covid-19 patients die while on their way to the hospital bathroom because they have to remove their oxygen masks before accessing the bathroom. Some simply don't have the physical strength to make it to the loo and back. An investment in these inexpensive conveniences may save more lives than spending on pricey manufactured ventilators which may or may not function.'

In Mission Save Lives, all deans and medical superintendents were mandated to ensure proper supply of medicines—antivirals, steroids, antibiotics, life-saving drugs and so on. While the efficacy of plasma therapy in treating Covid-19 is still disputed, there are individual cases where the therapy has shown results. 'Plasma banks were created in all hospitals under Mission Save Lives,' explains Chahal. 'That is when we found that plasma, contrary to some medical advice, was working well. I must narrate a small story of Aseem Gupta, a senior IAS officer. This officer was our secretary, energy. He contracted Covid-19 and was admitted to Lilavati Hospital. Aseem called me one day saying he was not feeling well and was very apprehensive. He had a great deal of anxiety. I told him not to worry. I would monitor his condition every day. The next day, he was taken to the ICU and put on a ventilator. He again told me he was fearful. I calmed him down and said we would take care of him.

'For the next 41 days, he was in the hospital. One evening, I got a message from his doctor that Assam may not survive. I had given him my word. So that day I called an emergency meeting of all the doctors. They said that the last resort was to give Aseem a plasma transfusion. His blood group was A+. One of the doctors called me and said they had plasma for AB+ and AB+ blood groups and it would work on A+ too. I told them I did not want to take any chances and wanted only A+ plasma for him. Ultimately, we got this plasma from JJ Hospital. The moment we gave him the plasma, he started recovering. Today he is fine and working. Every time we meet, he says you saved my life. After this I realised, despite contrasting medical opinions, the importance of plasma in treating Covid-19. We decided to create plasma banks in all hospitals. This too, became a part of Mission Save Lives.'

Chahal cites another case that occurred around the same time. A senior IAS officer, Idzes Angmo Kundan, who was an additional municipal commissioner in the MCGM several years ago, became critical at Breach Candy Hospital. She too, was given plasma and she too recovered. Now a number of hospitals have a plasma licence, says Chahal.

Under Mission Save Lives it was imperative that the reason for death was known. 'It shouldn't be that somebody had been recorded as having died due to Covid-19 but the real reason of death may be unknown,' Chahal points out. 'There should be a proper audit regarding the death of the person. From this we can learn the real reason for a fatality. By learning, we are able to save lives. So a death audit is conducted by the MCGM for every death. Whether medical or non-medical, a protocol is being followed based on medical/video recording. We decided that this mission should also be applicable to all private hospitals and private nursing homes which come under the jurisdiction of the MCGM. All the deans of major hospitals, medical superintendents of peripheral hospitals and the deans and the medical superintendents of government hospitals were instructed that the mission must be followed in the right spirit so as to save the life of every hospitalised Covid-19 patient. A weekly death audit report was to be submitted to the MCGM every Friday at 5.00 pm by the concerned deans and medical superintendents.

'We emphasised that the IAS officers appointed to monitor major hospitals should ensure that the above guidelines are strictly followed by all hospitals falling under our jurisdiction. This was additional work given to them by the order that I had earlier passed. Any non-compliance was to be brought to the notice of the municipal commissioner immediately. All private hospitals and nursing homes under the MCGM were asked to devise accurate mechanisms to achieve the objectives laid down under Mission Save Lives.'

Chahal said strict observance was necessary, given the severity of the second wave of Covid-19: 'The MCGM undertook surprise and random visits to inspect private premises and government hospitals to verify whether they had put the Mission Save Lives guidelines into action. To ensure this we created special squads. We had very clearly informed the private hospitals that there would be random visits. This mission did not involve any expenditure, it simply involved a certain amount of application, taking care of small issues and tightening the nuts and bolts. The death rate fell from 8 per cent to 7 per cent, then 6 per cent, then 5 per cent, then 4 per cent and we stabilised at 3.9 per cent at the end of 2020. By the beginning of 2022, the death rate in Mumbai had fallen to below 0.5 per cent.'

Writing in a philosophical vein on the cusp of the second wave, *Hindustan Times* editor-in-chief R. Sukumar noted[29]:

> 'Beyond the numbers, history will record the events of 2020 and 2021 along three dimensions: scientific, government, and individual. The scientific response to Covid-19 has been staggering in its speed and ingenuity. All previous records for vaccine development have been broken, not once, not twice, not three times, but several times over. A clutch of repurposed drugs and some new ones are now available to treat Covid-19. Death and hospitalisation rates have progressively reduced (with some exceptions). Science is winning.

[29] 1 March, 2021.

'The response of governments has been mixed—not surprising because of the scale and the complexity of the problem and the speed with which the disease emerged, and not surprising because governments have traditionally had an uneasy relationship with science and data, the only two things that should have, in ideal circumstances, driven their response to the pandemic. The Swedish, firm believers in science, seemed to turn their back on it in a strategy that was initially praised, then criticised, then acclaimed again, and finally debunked. For the record, I insisted all along that it was the wrong approach (not out of prescience but the understanding that when it came to pandemics, science could never be wrong). Still, while there were missteps (and there continue to be), and governments could have performed better than they did, and taken smarter decisions, they could just as easily have done worse on both counts. I just hope their experience with the pandemic has made governments realise what really matters (in this case, to repeat myself, science and data).

'Meanwhile, people adapted—to no jobs or those that paid less than they did before the pandemic; to constantly wearing masks; to social distancing, isolation, and quarantines; to not dining out or travelling; to working from home (or not working from home); to studying from home; and to many other things that would have seemed strange just a year ago. And so, scientists shone, governments faltered to varying degrees, and the rest of us, well, did what we do best—we coped.'

Coping with the pandemic is what the country did, with varying degrees of success. While the second wave was devastating, Professor Arvind Panagariya of Columbia University and former vice-chairman of NITI Aayog took stock[30] as the pandemic raged across India in the spring and summer of 2021:

> 'At the end of one year since the onset of the Covid-19 crisis, India can take pride in its accomplishments in several areas. First, at 11.9 per 1,00,000 individuals, the death rate due to Covid-19 stands at the lowest in India among the 20 most affected countries. The corresponding rate in the Czech Republic, the country with the highest death rate in this group, is 235.8. India fares almost equally well in terms of deaths as per cent of total infections. With its value at 1.4 per cent, it ranks 19th among the 20 most affected countries. Only Turkey in this group does better than India with a case-fatality ratio of 1.0 per cent.
>
> 'Second, India has done better than its peers in handling the economy. With the US and many European countries committing themselves to mega fiscal transfers, the pressure on the government in India to do the same was immense. But it recognised that with the movement of people outside their homes highly restricted, fiscal transfers could not translate into effective demand. And even if they could, with missing workers and broken input-supply chains, supply response to increased effective demand would have been lacking.'
>
> Panagariya added[31]: 'The first and foremost step towards averting another Covid-19 wave is much larger and faster investment in vaccine manufacturing. Assuming necessary raw materials are available, the objective should be to boost production capacity. Bharat Biotech need not be the only manufacturer of the vaccine. Production licences may be given to other credible and qualified manufacturers. If necessary, the government must use public funds to buy full ownership of the

[30]The *Times of India*, 1 April 2021.

[31]The *Times of India*, 28 April 2021.

patent on Covaxin at a reasonable price from Bharat Biotech. It should then mobilise multiple manufacturers to go full speed ahead. It should also invest in rapid expansion of other vaccines.

'A key reason why the United States has been able to move ahead rapidly with vaccination, barring a hiatus in between, is that its government invested heavily in de-risking vaccine research, trials and manufacturing early on. According to a paper by Chad Bown and Thomas Bollyky, the government began assisting vaccine manufacturers financially as early as February 2020. By 12 March 2021, it had committed more than $20 billion on clinical trials, manufacturing and future purchases of vaccine doses. Of this, more than $15 billion had been invested even before President Joe Biden took office.

'In an article published on 7 January 2021, I had recommended that India invest $8-10 billion in public money in vaccines. My argument then was that with the economy losing several billion dollars each week to Covid-19, we would more than recoup this investment through a speedier full restoration of economic activity. To this, we may add the benefit of saving tens of thousands of lives should there be another wave of infections.'

India's successful vaccination rollout soon silenced doubting Thomases. As the world's largest vaccine maker, India obviously had a key role to play in the global pandemic. Rhythm Kaul pointed[32] this out succintly:

'In less than a year since the vaccine development process began, India started manufacturing two shots—Serum Institute of India's (SII) Covishield and Bharat Biotech's Covaxin—not only for inoculation within the country, but also for shipping to countries abroad, a feat that underlined India's superlative

[32]*Hindustan Times*, 2 March 2021.

vaccine manufacturing capacity. The country, the world's largest vaccine maker by volume, supplies at least 60 per cent of all shots sold around the world.'

The Covid-19 pandemic, deep into its second year, took a heavy toll of health workers. The MCGM lost over 340 employees; nearly 10,000 became Covid-positive. Vaccinations helped, but inoculating the entire adult population of India—nearly a billion people—with two doses each obviously took time. Meanwhile, fatalities among frontline workers increased. An assistant commissioner in charge of H-East Ward passed away. One chief engineer too caught the infection and died. Several other MCGM engineers died. More than 115 BEST drivers lost their lives.

The second wave was cruel. It hit the middle class and the daily wage earners with equal ferocity. 'Covid is a long-drawn-out fight, it may go on for years,' Chahal reiterates. 'The first thing we should do is help our workers. So we did a couple of things. One, I decided to increase the financial packages of our employees. Those engaged in Covid work didn't have trains to board. They had to travel by taxis to report for work. The MCGM needed 100 per cent attendance, but with no suburban trains running for a major duration of the pandemic, how could we have expected a sweeper or a ward boy to come to our office from his home in a faraway suburb of Bhiwandi or Kalyan? So we started giving ₹300 per day as an honorary stipend to all MCGM workers. They could now travel by taxis as they were getting an extra ₹300 per day apart from their regular salary. We started running point-to-point buses from the suburbs to CSMT and Bandra stations.

'We increased the stipend to ₹600 per day for medical staff like nurses who were in the first, second or third year of their studies. We started paying them what a qualified nurse would get. We increased the stipend of doctors doing their residency. The central government had announced an insurance policy for Covid warriors. Doctors and nurses would get insurance of ₹50 lakh each. But when our people, like a BEST bus driver, died of Covid, I found that they did not fit into any of these definitions—they were neither doctors nor working in a hospital. Though they died of Covid while working for slum dwellers, the central government did not recognise them as Covid warriors or even as health workers or hospital workers.

'We therefore announced a policy of ₹50 lakh cash compensation for every employee of the MCGM who passed away directly or indirectly as a result of Covid-19, but who did not fit into the central government's insurance policy scheme. This was a major step. Although I passed this order in June 2020, I made it retrospective as of 1 March 2020. The order applies to every employee of the MCGM who has passed away while working for Covid-19. He could be a sweeper in a hospital or a health worker living in a slum, but his family gets ₹50 lakh irrespective of stature. No categorisation, no slabs. All BEST bus drivers were covered. BEST is a part of the MCGM. We proudly claim that we are the only civic body in the country with this cash compensation scheme. Fortunately, because of our strong financial position and our reserves, we can afford it, but this has been a game changer in raising the morale of our health workers, frontline workers and all MCGM employees. We also ensured that after receiving ₹50 lakh, a member of the affected family got a permanent job in the MCGM. Though we have lost so many employees in the fight against Covid-19, the morale of our staff remains high.'

Meanwhile, Mission Zero was executed by the MCGM to bring Covid-19 under total control in the city. Says Chahal: 'Over 50 mobile dispensaries and more than 100 private doctors were deployed in partnership with Bharati Jain Sangathana, MCHI-CREDAI and the Melinda and Bill Gates Foundation. We all joined hands and recruited 100 private doctors outside our rolls. They, in turn, brought in 50 mobile dispensaries. The purpose was to control the spread of the virus in 7 of 24 wards from where more than 50 per cent of Covid cases were emerging daily.

'It was decided to fight the menace with the help of NGO participation and implement our chase the virus policy more aggressively. As infectivity rose, in Mumbai, we decided to start moving people in the ratio of 1:20. For every one Covid-positive patient, we picked up 20 people, rather than 15 as we had done earlier. Anyone with close contact with a patient was put in quarantine. Meanwhile, the 50 mobile dispensaries entered the containment zones of these 7 vulnerable wards and acted as mobile hospitals there. They conducted RT-PCR tests, antigen tests, and took comorbid people to the hospital.'

During the city's Mission Zero initiative, testing labs were told to employ additional manpower. For every ambulance, one health worker in a PPE kit took swabs on the spot at people's homes. The MCGM paid the lab technicians' salaries, though they were lab employees. 'The mobile dispensaries became like a moving RT-PCR lab,' says Chahal. 'That is how the testing rate went up, especially in the slums and chawls. The mobile dispensary carried medicines, oxygen and a qualified doctor. Such mobile dispensaries will be useful to complete the vaccination drive in the coming months for both adults and children.'

The lethal second wave underscored the importance of Jumbo field hospitals. 'We found that people were initially reluctant to go to these Jumbos, thinking that they are created in the open and we will die there,' recalls Chahal. 'Everyone wanted a hospital like KEM, Sion and Nair, no one wanted a Jumbo. To put up 9,000 beds in Jumbos was a massive challenge of staffing. While we had already recruited senior doctors for the Jumbos, as cases rose, even more challenging was recruiting senior specialist doctors and interventionists specifically for Jumbo ICUs. So we came up with a novel idea. We had received feedback that a number of private hospitals and small nursing homes in Mumbai were still lying shut. Their doctors were sitting at home. These doctors used to run ICUs and upto 50-bed nursing homes. We decided to float a tender and asked these doctors if together, as a group, they could run our Jumbo ICUs on an outsourced basis. From a ward boy to a nurse, a specialist doctor and a super-specialist doctor—we would pay them per bed per day. We also gave a 50 per cent bed occupancy guarantee.

'We got responses from four different groups of doctors. We received the best bid at ₹7,000 per bed per day. For the ICU beds within the Jumbos, the medicines and equipment would be ours, but all medical personnel, starting from the ward boy to the super-specialist doctor, would be theirs. They provided 100 per cent staffing. All the infrastructure was ours. Super-specialists doctors get ₹5 lakh a month, the younger ones get ₹1 lakh a month, aand nurses get ₹2,000 per day for ICUs. Additional Commissioner Sanjeev Jaiswal did an outstanding job and organised everything. From idea to execution, it took just 15 days. We had told the doctors that all medical council guidelines to run an ICU within a Jumbo must be adhered to. No one should complain that the ICUs are not fully and completely staffed. If any expert from anywhere in the country inspects them, we should be able to show him that we are following MCA guidelines for ICUs on the of ratio of doctors, ratio of specialists, ratio of nurses, and ratio of ward boys. Super-specialist staff to run the ICUs functioning within the Jumbos would otherwise have been impossible to find in those critical times.

There still remained a perception among affluent patients that government-run hospitals and the 11 outsourced Jumbo field hospitals were not as clean and medically competent as private hospitals. Chahal strongly contested this. He decided to do something about it: 'I came up with the idea of starting a mentorship programmes for the Jumbos. For the Worli Dome Jumbo, Breach Candy Hospital and Bombay Hospital acted as mentors. For BKC 1 and 2, Lilavati and Hinduja Hospitals were designated mentors. For the Mulund Jumbo, Wockhart and Fortis Hospitals were mentors. For the NESCO Jumbo, Nanavati and Life Care Hospitals were selected as mentors. All Jumbo field hospitals were linked with major private hospitals in their vicinity. In order to provide quality healthcare to patients, 38 private medical consultants attached to major private hospitals agreed to provide their services to the MCGM's Jumbo field hospitals through telemedicine and personal visits on weekends.

'The following role was assigned to these 38 consulting doctors: One, to mentor doctors in the linked Jumbo facility by teleconference and consultation with a specialist in the private hospital in order to guide the treating doctor of the Jumbo hospital. This was an honorary arrangement. Two, to visit the linked Jumbo hospital once a week to impart advice to the treating doctors. That, in turn, provided a great deal of assurance to the patients. Three, to empower the deans of Jumbo Covid hospitals to utilise these consultant services at their respective facilities.

'The top private doctors who visited the Jumbo facilities included Dr Zarir Udwadia, Dr Pravin Amin, Dr Gautam Bhansali, Dr Pratibha Singhal, Dr Arya Bansal, Dr Hemant Thacker and Dr Pratit Samdani. This programme is ongoing in 2022 as we strengthen our healthcare infrastructure. The Jumbos have private rooms, their own pathology labs, nursing stations, resting rooms for doctors, private consultation rooms and rooms for yoga and meditation.

'The mentorship scheme, the outsourcing model, getting more patients into 5-star Jumbo field hospitals to take the pressure off other hospitals—these have made Mumbai's 11 Jumbos a unique healthcare model both in India and globally. While they may seem under-utilised at times, in 2022 they have added to our capacity to deal with new viruses, including the Omicron variant and future mutants.' Operational Jumbos were reduced from 11 to 9 and then, as the third wave abated by March 2022, even these were used as vaccination hubs, including for children aged 12–14.

Beyond the immediate task of healing lives and livelihoods in wave after wave of the pandemic, the focus shifted to enhancing India's overall healthcare infrastructure. Sandhya Venkateswaran described the challenge[33]:

> 'The pandemic disrupted life, livelihoods, education and health like little else in recent history. The world found innovations and adaptations to minimise some of the disruptions for some people, but not all. Healthcare disruptions, less amenable to home-based solutions, ranged across a very broad continuum—a shift in health-seeking behaviour, limitations in health infrastructure, difficulties in outreach to community members, lack of availability of human resources and interruptions in supply chains. Not all of these were limited to the context of the pandemic—some have pre-existed but got magnified in the context of the pandemic.
>
> 'Covid-19 saw healthcare workers diverted to the much-needed task of preventing and dealing with infections, taking them away from their regular tasks, and thus further reducing the availability of healthcare workers. Healthcare facilities were deployed for testing and treating patients, but this made them unavailable for regular services. Supply chains were disrupted due to lockdowns. When health facilities were functioning, citizens were either fearful or unable to travel to them or

[33]*Hindustan Times*, 10 March 2021.

were unaware that facilities were functioning. All this led to significant disruption in the provision of essential health services such as routine immunisation, testing and treating tuberculosis (TB) patients, maternal and child healthcare and nutrition-related interventions.

'But India is no stranger to innovation. A few months into the pandemic, there were a variety of interventions which sought to address some of these barriers related to health human resources, demand for and access to services, and provision to the last mile. Innovations were found in at least four categories—leveraging technology, leveraging community platforms, strengthening frontline workers and augmenting supply chains.

'India saw many innovations rolled out, although not necessarily at scale and most not evaluated for impact. Based on rigorous impact evaluations, there is potential for scale and convergence. It is not that this potential is not recognised by the government. The introduction of telemedicine guidelines and the launch of the National Digital Health Mission provide a foundation for greater leverage of the digital platform. Admittedly, limited internet penetration in rural India, gender disparity in internet usage, and concerns about data privacy and data-sharing ethics limit the impact of digital platforms. But an increasing focus on health technology platforms can address, to some extent, the needs of information, triaging, counselling, consultation, scheduling visits, home delivery of drugs, and remote follow-up, reducing some of the demand- and supply-side challenges.'

Global media too finally focused its attention on Mumbai's rapid response to crises. Bloomberg's Dhwani Pandya and P.R. Saniyal recaptured[34], to drive home their point, a pivotal moment in Mumbai's battle against Covid-19:

> 'At midnight on 17 April, as a deadly new wave of the coronavirus overwhelmed India, Mumbai's Municipal Commissioner Iqbal Singh Chahal learned that 6 hospitals in his city would run out of oxygen within hours—putting the lives of 168 patients at risk. Amid the ensuing scramble, the patients were rushed to the temporary hospitals Chahal's team had set up during the city's first wave in 2020. He hadn't dismantled the facilities even when cases dipped. Unlike most Indian hospitals that relied on cylinders, they had been equipped with pipes that supplied oxygen directly to patients' beds. All 168 survived.
>
> 'That night—which Chahal described as the scariest he's ever had—offers a look at tactics India's financial capital used to quell its outbreak faster, and with fewer casualties, than other parts of the country. Chahal attributes the city's successes partly to a decentralised system his team set up during the first wave, which included neighbourhood war rooms to manage cases by locality. He's also made vast changes to the way the city sourced and used its medical oxygen, creating emergency stocks and tracking systems for tankers. So, even as families around India desperately pleaded for supplies on social media, Mumbai's patients reported fewer problems. With a population of 15 million spread across glistening skyscrapers, apartment complexes and sprawling slums, Mumbai is the world's second-most densely packed city, according to data from the United Nations. About 32,000 people are crammed in per square kilometre. That makes lessons from India's financial capital

[34]Bloomberg, 21 May 2021.

particularly valuable as fears grow about outbreaks in other crowded places from Bangkok to Kathmandu.'

On 1 May 2021, when Covid-19 was creating havoc in the country, the BJP's Member of Parliament Subramanian Swamy tweeted: 'Uddhav Thackeray government needs a small pat on the back (big pat if trend continues) for lowering the coronavirus infections rate in Mumbai. I believe even hospitals are now in a better shape.' Says Chahal: 'Showing a big heart, CM Thackeray messaged me, "Credit goes to your hard work". 'Supriya Sule, Member of Parliament and daughter of Sharad Pawar, messaged "You are not Iqbal Chahal. You are superman Chahal". ' The pandemic, meanwhile, raged worldwide.

Covid-19 has infected several hundred million people globally and killed over 5 million. Those are the official figures. The actual number of fatalities from the coronavirus pandemic are obviously far higher. Scientists and researchers continue to ask the question. Where did the Covid-19 virus originate? Abhilash Gaur made some thoughtful observations[35]: 'The leading theory is that it was a bat virus that somehow learnt to infect humans. But how that happened is a question that divides scientists. The vocal majority says the crossover from bats to humans happened naturally. Those who suggest that the virus may have escaped from a Chinese research lab are labelled batty conspiracy theorists. But this minority is making itself heard. Several recent articles in reputed publications challenge the view that a lab leak is out of the question.

'Mind you, they are not saying China made the virus with malicious intent. They are not calling it a biological weapon. All they are saying is that for the past several years, a big lab in

[35]*The Times of India.*

Wuhan has been tweaking coronaviruses—the family to which the Covid virus belongs—to see which ones can cause a future pandemic. What's wrong with investigating the possibility of an accidental leak from this lab, they ask. The lab in question is the Wuhan Institute of Virology (WIV), and is "around 10 miles (16 kilometres) from the site of the initial outbreak in Wuhan," Dr Norman Paradis, a professor of medicine at Dartmouth College, wrote in the science journal *Undark*. Behind its low red-brick facade, the WIV "runs the world's leading effort geared toward collecting wild coronaviruses from that region, and they are reported to have tinkered with the wild viruses to develop potent new strains," he added.

'Another *Undark* article by Charles Schmidt that was republished by *MIT Technology Review*, says scientists at the institute nudge viruses to change so that they can infect humans and become more infectious or lethal. It's a way to prepare for something that might happen naturally years from now. Nicholson Baker described it in detail earlier this year in *New York* magazine: "Over the past few decades, scientists have... learned how to trick viruses, coronaviruses in particular... into moving quickly from one species of animal to another or from one type of cell culture to another."

'The closest relative of SARS-CoV-2 is a bat virus called RaTG13, which WIV scientists collected from a cave in Yunnan province in 2013. The two viruses are 96.2 per cent similar, and the US State Department says WIV has been experimenting on RaTG13 since 2016.'

R. Sukumar has followed the Covid-19 pandemic closely. On 14 May 2021 he wrote in the *Hindustan Times* on the likely origin of the coronavirus, WHO's dilatory response and China's opacity:

> 'A report released on Wednesday on what went wrong with the world's (and the World Health Organization's) response to the coronavirus disease doesn't have any surprising revelations. The report, prepared by the Independent Panel for Pandemic Preparedness and Response (IPPPR) that was set up after various WHO members demanded it, lists some suggestions on preparing for the next pandemic, including the creation of a Global Health Threats Council (its members will be heads of state, and also from civil society and the private sector), and an International Pandemic Financing Facility which will be funded by rich countries to the tune of $5-10 billion a year, and which will help countries prepare for or manage pandemics, that, while not entirely new (again), do seem like good moves. The best time to prepare for the next pandemic is soon after seeing the current one off.
>
> 'The report terms February 2020 the lost month—if the WHO had acted then, or if the countries had, the trajectory of the pandemic is likely to have been very different from one that has, over the 17 months since 1 January 2020, caused 161 million infections and 3.34 million deaths around the world. The actual numbers of the infected and the dead are likely to be much higher. On 14 January 2020, the WHO claimed, on the basis of investigations carried out by Chinese health authorities, that there was "no clear human-to-human transmission". A week later, it changed its position, and said there was possibility of "sustained" human-to-human transmission. It delayed declaring a public health emergency till 31 January, and terming the outbreak a pandemic till 11 March. It wasn't until June that the multilateral health agency would issue a proper advisory on masks (which it did not recommend till then).

And while it did accept the possibility that the virus could be airborne last year, it wasn't until earlier this year that it changed its guidelines to include this. Most worryingly, through this period, the WHO has made no headway in figuring out the origin of the virus which first appeared in Wuhan, China.

'The debate over whether the virus was made in a lab, or evolved in nature, is ongoing, and more research is needed before a definite answer can be provided. In early May 2021, science writer Nicholas Wade summarised the research so far, laying out the cases for and against either scenario. Wade's article, published in *Medium*, leans towards the lab argument, but it isn't a conspiracy theory. Instead, he presents a cogent scientific argument built around three strands.

'One, provenance, or how, if the virus was naturally found in the famous horseshoe bats of Yunnan, it travelled all the way to Wuhan, at least 1,500 kilometres away; two, evolution, or how the SARS-CoV-2 virus, which causes the coronavirus disease, came fully evolved to optimally target humans, unlike the Sars-CoV virus, responsible for South Asia Respiratory Syndrome, that evolved over time to become efficient at targeting humans; and finally, the unique furin cleavage site that the virus possesses, not found in other beta coronaviruses, and activated by an enzyme, furin, commonly found in human cells. The furin cleavage site has figured in this column previously because it is truly unique. The spike protein of Sars-CoV-2 has three parts—S1, S2, and a cleavage site at the boundary. Furin cleaves the two, and the S1 site then attaches to the ACE receptor (also found commonly on the surface of human cells), a binding that facilitates the entry of the viral protein into the human cell. You can read Wade's piece (I'd recommend it) at nicholaswade.medium.com.'

This is what Wade concludes in his lengthy and well-researched article in The *Bulletin of the Atomic Scientists* that was widely quoted globally:

> 'It's documented that researchers at the Wuhan Institute of Virology were doing gain-of-function experiments designed to make coronaviruses infect human cells and humanised mice. This is exactly the kind of experiment from which a SARS2-like virus could have emerged. The researchers were not vaccinated against the viruses under study, and they were working in the minimal safety conditions of a BSL-2 laboratory. So escape of a virus would not be at all surprising. In all of China, the pandemic broke out on the doorstep of the Wuhan institute. The virus was already well adapted to humans, as expected for a virus grown in humanised mice. It possessed an unusual enhancement, a furin cleavage site, which is not possessed by any other known SARS-related beta-coronavirus, and this site included a double arginine codon also unknown among beta-coronaviruses. What more evidence could you want, aside from the presently unobtainable lab records documenting SARS2's creation?
>
> 'As may now be obvious, there are many people who have reason not to talk about it. The list is led, of course, by the Chinese authorities. But virologists in the United States and Europe have no great interest in igniting a public debate about the gain-of-function experiments that their community has been pursuing for years. Nor have other scientists stepped forward to raise the issue. Government research funds are distributed on the advice of committees of scientific experts drawn from universities. Anyone who rocks the boat by raising awkward political issues runs the risk that their grant will not be renewed and their research career will be ended.

Maybe good behaviour is rewarded with the many perks that slosh around the distribution system. And if you thought that Andersen and Daszak might have blotted their reputation for scientific objectivity after their partisan attacks on the lab escape scenario, look at the second and third names on this list of recipients of an $82 million grant announced by the National Institute of Allergy and Infectious Diseases in August 2020.

'Fauci is a longtime public servant who served with integrity under President Trump and has resumed leadership in the Biden administration in handling the COVID-19 epidemic. Congress, no doubt understandably, may have little appetite for hauling him over the coals for the apparent lapse of judgment in funding gain-of-function research in Wuhan. To these serried walls of silence must be added that of the mainstream media. To my knowledge, no major newspaper or television network has yet provided readers with an in-depth news story on the lab escape scenario, such as the one you have just read, although some have run brief editorials or opinion pieces. One might think that any plausible origin of a virus that has killed 3 million people would merit a serious investigation. Or that the wisdom of continuing gain-of-function research, regardless of the virus's origin, would be worth some probing. Or that the funding of gain-of-function research by the NIH and NIAID during a moratorium on such funding would bear investigation. What accounts for the media's apparent lack of curiosity?'

While China stonewalls investigation of the origin of the coronavirus, world opinion has turned sharply against it. *The Economist,* citing a new Danish television documentary, rightly asked[36] for a "proper investigation" into the origin of Covid-19: 'The virus mystery,' broadcast on 12 August 2021, drew uncommonly wide attention for a Danish television documentary. That was because it featured Peter Ben Embarek, an expert on food security and zoonotic diseases, casting doubt on the conclusions of a "joint study" on the origins of the covid-19 pandemic carried out earlier this year under the auspices of the World Health Organization (WHO). Dr Ben Embarek was the senior who figure who went to China as part of that study.

'In March, the joint study reported that it was "extremely unlikely" that the virus had been released in a laboratory accident. Dr Ben Embarek revealed that this conclusion did not come from a balanced assessment of all the relevant evidence but from a steadfast refusal by the Chinese members of the joint study to support anything stronger. Indeed they only allowed even that minimal assessment on the condition that the report did not call for further investigation into the question.

'He also pointed out that the idea that the point of spillover was someone collecting bat samples for research purposes belongs in the "likely" basket, along with other human interactions with wild bats.

'Problems in the joint study had long been clear. Within the WHO one source describes it as "riddled with compromises and sloppiness». Tedros Adhanom Ghebreyesus, the WHO's director-general, was uneasy about the way it was carried out. He pushed back at the marginalisation of the lab-leak hypothesis, particularly when the final report was released in March. He has since called for further investigations into it, as well as into other possibilities.

'The further unravelling of the joint study matters because, more than a year and a half after the Covid-19 outbreak in Wuhan, a city in Hubei, was first recognised as the work of a new pathogen, there has

[36]*The Economist*, 21 August 2021.

been nothing like a thorough international investigation of how that pathogen, SARS-CoV-2, got into humans and spread around the world. The pandemic's death toll stands at 9 m-18 m, according to a model which *The Economist* has built on the basis of excess-mortality reports and other indicators. The question of how it started matters both for the relatives of the dead and for those who wish to prevent such an outbreak from happening again. China's efforts to stop the world from answering it are both shabby and, to an extent, self-defeating. The more the truth seems hidden, the more it seems suspicious.'

Meanwhile, as the scientific and medical debate on the origin of SARS-CoV-2 intensifies, Chahal remains focused on the job at hand. Having weathered a particularly ferocious monsoon season in 2020—floods, storms and cyclones—during the first wave of the pandemic, Mumbai was hit in 2021 by another unusual weather system. For Chahal it was déjà vu. Nearly a year after cyclone Narsarga had struck Mumbai, cyclone Tauktae swirled over the city in May 2021. Again, three vulnerable Jumbos had to be evacuated.

One report[37] noted graphically:

> 'As Cyclone Tauktae made its way northward along the coast of Karnataka and Maharashtra on Sunday evening, the MCGM scrambled to move patients from Covid centres to government hospitals in the city. Until late in the evening, a total 603 Covid-19 patients had been moved out of three Jumbo facilities in the city, including 243 from the BKC facility, 184 from the Dahisar facility, and 176 from Mulund. Some were discharged, the rest were admitted to hospitals run by the state government and the civic body. Mumbai saw 44 per

[37] *Indian Express,* 17 May 2021.

> cent of its entire average June rainfall in one day on 9 June 2021 and 84 per cent of the season's rainfall in 9 days. From 17-19 July 2021, the city experienced 70 per cent of the average July rainfall in 3 days.'

Fortunately, the rest of the 2021 monsoon season passed off uneventfully even though the total rainfall crossed 3,500 mm—a record again after 2020. Chahal turned his attention to a common, but largely ignored, complaint among hospitalised and quarantined patients with mild symptoms: loneliness. Patients have little or no contact with family or friends. Chahal thought of an innovative way to alleviate the problem. He calls it the iPad concept. 'The consul general of South Africa had met me and I told her about this iPad concept,' he says. 'After going through the content detailing the concept, she sent me a message: "Thank you for availing yourself to meet me and for sharing the information. I have forwarded the entire note to my capital city (in South Africa) as a best practice example and I have told my capital city to follow this."

'We started a helpline here in association with M Power, an NGO run by Neerja Birla, wife of Aditya Birla Group chairman Kumar Mangalam Birla. She is doing great work addressing mental health issues, depression and psychological problems faced by citizens. The MCGM tied up with M Power and we started helplines for Covid patients. A number of patients who became Covid-negative later on, asymptomatic people who were suspected to have Covid, repeatedly called on the helplines saying that they were feeling depressed and even suicidal. We don't feel like continuing to live, they said, we are fed up of the lockdowns. When they were admitted to hospitals,they were completely isolated. Many were paranoid, thinking the worst, that they were not going to meet their families again.

'As a team we decided we must address this issue quickly. In one of our meetings it was agreed that Covid-19 is a peculiar pandemic where the affected patient gets totally isolated from the world. He is not able to see his wife, children, parents, brothers, sisters, and friends for days together. Sometimes there are instances where patients don't become Covid-negative for as long as 21 to 28 days. That is what brings upon the depression. A feeling of anxiety and loneliness prevails.

'To tackle this issue, we came up with an idea. We decided that for at least the MCGM hospitals, whether they are our Jumbos or KEM, Nair, Sion, etc., we would make use of the internet facilities there. All hospital systems today work on WiFi technology—ICU equipment, pathology labs, etc. We decided to purchase a large number of iPads: one iPad for 5 patients. We spent ₹1.5 crore to procure these iPads. It would not be a waste of money because when the pandemic finally ends, we will distribute the iPads to children in municipal schools free of cost. But now, with the iPads, non-ICU Covid patients could chat on audio and video calls with their families and friends.

'This idea became a great success because it immediately lifted patient morale. They could talk to and see their families every day. The family members too, were happy that the patient was being kept in 5-star Jumbo facilities and was well-looked-after there. Video calls could also be made by patients to mentor-doctors for advice on their medical reports and medication required. The notional value of addressing and curing the psychological problems of patients is priceless. The iPads not only helped relieve patients' isolation and anxiety, but helped in video conferencing and teleconferencing with specialist doctors. The South African consul general said they had tens of thousands of active cases in her country and she has adopted this iPad concept for hospitalised Covid patients there.'

As a palliative measure, this was another innovation in the long battle against Covid-19. But sterner challenges lay ahead.

SEVEN

MASS PUBLIC CAMPAIGN

The first wave of the Covid-19 pandemic peaked in India's blistering summer of 2020, and then ebbed—or seemed to ebb—as winter approached. It would prove a false dawn. Guards were lowered. But Covid's deadly variants lay in wait as the country went back to work.

'By the first week of September 2020,' says Chahal, 'Covid was well under control. But Mumbai was still recording about 1,000 cases every day. This would multiply to over 10,000 cases a day in the city in April 2021. But back in September 2020, the situation was different. There were early signs that the first wave was finally, 7 months after it struck Mumbai, coming under control. We needed to keep up the pressure on all fronts—medical, preemption, health infrastructure and communications. The chief minister called me to his official residence Varsha for a meeting on evolving a mass advertising campaign to educate people on Covid-appropriate behaviour. The idea of launching a large-scale people's movement is very important. A number of peer-reviewed research studies had shown that a mask is a good shield against Covid. Even in a post-pandemic environment, masks should be worn when appropriate. In Japan, wearing a mask in public has been a habit for decades. Let me share my own experience.

'I visited Tokyo in July 2003 for some work. I boarded a train from the main station Shinjuku, close to where I was staying. I took the train to go to my destination in Tokyo. I was astonished to see that almost everybody in the train was wearing a mask. It was a packed train. There were possibly only 5-7 people without a mask among hundreds of passengers. I was wondering at that time, way back in 2003, why this was so. Now, nearly 20 years later, when I look back, I realise what a good habit the Japanese have. It partly explains why Japan has been spared large-scale Covid-19 cases and fatalities despite a surge in Tokyo and other cities in 2021 before and after the Olympic Games in August. The way Japan pulled off the Tokyo Olympics so successfully in the midst of a global pandemic is a tribute to the country's discipline and healthcare infrastructure. When a Covid monitoring team from the Union government came to assess the situation in Mumbai, we had highlighted the importance of face masks in fighting Covid-19. A vaccine was still not available at the time. This virus spreads like wildfire, wave after wave, surge after surge. A simple mask can help prevent the spread.

'In that crucial meeting at Varsha, I would give full credit to the CM, Uddhav Thackeray, whom I admire, for proposing a mask campaign, a mask movement. He said let us name this campaign in Marathi '*Maza Kutumb Mazi Jababdari*'. Kutumb means family. Jababdari means responsibility. We also translated it into English, 'My Family My Responsibility', and in Hindi, 'Mera Parivar Meri Jimmedari'. Over a period of two or three meetings in the first week of September, towards the end of the peak of the initial wave, we took some key decisions. I realised that this would be a unique campaign. No city in the world has ever created and launched a mass campaign where the local authority in charge of controlling the pandemic visits almost every home and every family. It was unprecedented.'

The MCGM decided to run the initial mass public campaign from 15 September to 15 November 2020. 'Once the concept was crystalised,' Chahal says, 'I did a social media broadcast to 300 editors and principal correspondents of newspapers, online news portals and TV networks all over the country and abroad on 11 September. The MCGM issued a press note on the same day explaining the campaign's objectives. We said we need to learn to live with the coronavirus. Once a virus enters our system, it does not go away forever—whether it is tuberculosis, polio, leprosy, dengue or malaria. It may happen that the coronavirus will be in the ecosystem for a long time. We decided, therefore, that instead of saying we will eradicate Covid-19, we would say that we have to learn to live with this virus for years and educate people on how best to remain safe.

'Initially, the campaign was driven by the MCGM, but it should now become a part of our lives. Until we get complete control over the pandemic, it is important to make some changes in our lifestyle, going beyond the use of masks, maintaining physical distancing and using sanitisers. It is necessary, after the second wave, the third wave and all the succeeding waves that may come, to adopt some changes in our personal, family and public lives. In accordance, My Family My Responsibility was a campaign aimed at spreading the message of dealing with the crisis in a holistic way with a long-term perspective going well beyond 2021.'

The campaign was implemented with broad participation: politicians, citizens and NGOs. The objective was to motivate more and more people to adopt a new lifestyle for effective Covid control with Covid-appropriate behaviour. To counter future waves and intra-wave surges of the coronavirus, effective healthcare education to control the spread of Covid-19 in the long-term is clearly imperative. Under the mass public campaign, volunteers appointed by the public health department of the MCGM reached out to nearly each family in areas under the civic body's jurisdiction, going door-to-door.

After successive waves of Covid-19 cascaded across rural and urban India in spurts through 2021 and 2022, preventive measures became critical. The mass contact campaign in Mumbai provided referral treatment to people with comorbidities such as diabetes, heart disease, kidney failure and obesity. Volunteers met each family twice during the campaign to curtail the spread of Covid-19 and its variants. Health workers urged all members of the family to take necessary care and be vigilant to avoid even inadvertent mistakes. Citizens were informed in detail about the important steps that should be taken to win the battle against Covid-19. The three-pronged approach to take preventive steps in personal, family and public life were spelt out in an advisory note:

1. Maintain a safe distance of at least 2 metres between each other.
2. Use masks regularly and properly.
3. Wash your hands frequently and use sanitisers properly.

The advisory added that all citizens must follow this three-pronged approach. Other important steps that needed to be included in the citizens' daily lives were set out clearly:

1. At an individual level, measure body temperature and oxygen levels every morning.
2. Always use a mask. Do not remove it or wear it under the nose. Family members should ensure that each member of the family is taking due care.
3. Do not touch your face or mask often.
4. After using a single-use mask, spray sanitiser and then cut it into pieces in order to prevent reuse.

The MCGM received information that the Mumbai police had raided one area where several lakh used masks were found. These were being packed and readied to be sold again. It was vital, therefore, to cut used masks into pieces so that they cannot be reused.

Other pointers in the advisory included instructions to counter future waves of the pandemic and not letting the guard down:

1. Carry a bottle of sanitiser and use it as often and when needed.
2. Keep your hands clean by washing them frequently with soap.
3. Carry a clean handkerchief. If you have a cough and cold, use a mask and a handkerchief.
4. Reusable masks should be washed daily.
5. Family members should use different types of masks or mark their respective masks to avoid confusion. Do not share masks.
6. Include vitamin-rich food in your diet.
7. Avoid talking while eating food.
8. Include more vegetables and protein-rich food in your meals.
9. Ensure adequate meals and sleep and practice yoga to build body immunity.
10. Always wear a mask while driving or travelling in a vehicle.
11. Talking to traffic police and other citizens without wearing masks increases the risk of infection. Therefore, it is important to wear masks at all times even while travelling.
12. Avoid confined environments, crowds and close contact with others.
13. Bathe and wash your clothes when you return home from office or outdoors.
14. Avoid visiting areas, cities, states, countries where Covid-19 is still leading to multiple positive cases.
15. Keep a note of the places you have visited and the people you have met if you have developed symptoms of Covid-19. This is very handy in high-risk contact tracing.

Guidelines at the family level were also issued to avoid reinfections. Many of these are relevant during surges but serve as useful guidance even after the pandemic abates, movie theatres open and schools resume.

Lowering one's guard again could set off a mini-surge of infections.

1. If a member of the family violates Covid-19 guidelines, it must be brought to his/her notice by other members of the family.
2. Always carry an oximeter to measure oxygen levels. Oxygen levels of each member of the family must be checked at regular intervals. An accurate record should be maintained.
3. Carry a thermometer or a thermal screening gun.
4. Special attention should be paid towards the health of children and the elderly.
5. Ensure that these members of the family who have comorbidities take their medication regularly and maintain their immunity.
6. Where possible, sit beside each other instead of opposite each other while eating food with the family.
7. As far as possible, only one member of the family should go out for work.
8. All members must wear clean clothes every day. Do not reuse unwashed clothes.
9. Personal items such as mobile phones should not be exchanged among family members. Such items must also be kept clean.
10. Food parcels should not be left in the kitchen for long if ordered from outside.
11. Immediately cover dustbins after disposal of food containers and packets.
12. Vegetables and fruits should be cleaned before being used.
13. If a parcel ordered from outside contains non-perishable items, do not open the parcel for at least a day. Spray sanitiser on it and open it the next day.
14. Floors, kitchens and toilets should be cleaned regularly using disinfectants.

15. Indian-style toilets should be kept clean and the lid of western toilets must be kept shut while flushing. This is important.
16. Avoid meeting relatives and friends in large groups.
17. Family events and parties should be avoided. If unavoidable, follow government guidelines for Covid-19.

The corporation issued this advisory to housing societies and colonies. These too need to be followed even when Covid-19 infections have seemingly abated and social functions begun to be held.

1. Wear a mask while walking in society premises.
2. All residents must use sanitisers, masks and gloves while leaving the house.
3. Children and senior citizens should avoid stepping out of the house except for essential work during Covid-19 surges.
4. Maintain a distance of at least 6 feet while communicating with anybody in the society.
5. Avoid using common waiting rooms in societies.
6. Avoid touching door handles, elevators, railings, wall, and benches in the society premises.
7. Keep a small piece of paper in your hand while using the elevator. These pieces of paper must be disposed of immediately after use.
8. On returning home, wash your hands thoroughly with sanitiser and soap
9. No one from outside the society premises should be given direct access to your family without authorisation.
10. Ensure that temperature checking, oxygen checking and hand-washing facilities are available for outsiders, drivers, waste collectors, cleaners and other workers.
11. Arrangements should be made to keep ordered parcels in a safe place at the entrance of the society instead of receiving them directly at home.

12. Sanitise the parcel before taking it home.
13. Vehicles should be sanitised from inside before they leave the society's premises.
14. Display important contact numbers like nearby municipal health centres, hospitals and ward war rooms in the society's premises.

Many of these guidelines may appear excessively cautious when a wave has receded, but common sense should dictate precautions that are necessary in varying circumstances. Guidelines at shopping markets and malls remain in operation as well, given the unpredictability of Covid-19 and its latent infectivity even after multiple waves have ebbed.

1. Ensure that only one person goes out for shopping at a time, not the entire family.
2. Maintain a safe distance from others both inside and outside shops.
3. Do not enter a shop if it is crowded.
4. Take the stairs instead of the elevator if it is crowded. Do not touch the hand railings.
5. Avoid touching items on display in shops and malls.
6. Shop online as far as possible.
7. Shopkeepers should not allow customers not wearing a mask to enter.
8. Only a limited number of customers should be allowed to enter a shop, market or mall to maintain safe physical distance.
9. Arrangements to check body temperature and sanitisation should be made for all those entering a shop.
10. Limited number of staff/helpers should be appointed in shops, markets, and shopping complexes.

11. Risk of infection should be reduced by handling currency sparingly.

It was recommended that specific guidelines should be in operation at workplaces and offices as India gets used to working in the 'new normal.' Work from home (wfh) and work from anywhere (wfa) have created a new work paradigm. A hybrid model is being followed by several corporates, allowing certain categories of employees a flexible working protocol. Workplaces, though, need to treat safety as a priority as staff return to office in increasing numbers.

1. The office should be designed in such a way that there is a safe physical distance between all employees.
2. Employees should be called on alternate days and as needed.
3. Working hours should be staggered.
4. Equipment to check body temperature, oxygen levels and sanitisation should be available to all staff members.
5. Use video conferencing for meetings as far as possible.
6. Digital work should be adopted to minimise human contact.
7. Keep windows open in the office to make way for fresh air.
8. Avoid the use of air conditioning systems as far as possible.
9. Office/work tours should be avoided unless absolutely necessary.
10. Commute during less crowded hours.
11. Use a mask and sanitiser in office and sit at a safe distance from others.
12. Use a mask and sanitiser while travelling and at meetings in office.
13. Maintain a safe distance while interacting with visitors in office.

Guidelines for travelling by private and public vehicles are equally important:

1. Maintain silence while travelling by public transport.
2. Do not talk to fellow passengers unless necessary.
3. It is advisable to use a face shield along with a mask while travelling in public transportation, especially trains.
4. Avoid travelling by crowded vehicles; do not touch the door handles of the vehicle.

Some believe that such preventive advisories are unnecessary in a post-Covid world. That is a fallacy. There is no such thing as a post-Covid world. Future waves of the pandemic, as the virus continues to mutate, can strike anytime, anywhere, anyone, even after the full vaccination programme has been completed by 2022. As and when a pandemic becomes endemic, normalcy in life and at work will return, but caution must remain, the watchword.

'It is important to adopt all the above measures as a part of your lifestyle,' Chahal emphasises. 'Citizens need to comply with the guidelines and cooperate with the government to retain effective control over Covid-19.'

While alarmist projections can damage public morale, the threat of a new Covid-19 wave remains ever-present. The spike in cases in the United States despite a vaccination rollout, and the Omicron surge across the world, are examples of how swiftly, and without warning, the virus can return.

On cue, the *Times of India* front-paged this report on 23 August 2021:

> 'A committee of experts constituted under the National Institute of Disaster Management (NIDM) has warned of an imminent third wave of Covid and sought better medical preparedness for children who might be at similar risk as adults. The report of the committee, set up on the directions of the home ministry, has noted that "paediatric facilities—doctors, staff, equipment like ventilators, ambulances, etc. are nowhere close to what

may be required in case a large number of children become infected". The report has been submitted to the PMO.

'The report has called for prioritising vaccination among children with comorbidities and a special focus on those with disability. The vulnerability of children, as they haven't been vaccinated, has been discussed, with most experts being of the view that they are not prone to severe infections though they can pass the virus to others. Other estimates have said a third wave, seen to be the result of renewed mobility, may prove to be less severe than the second.

'The study: "Third Wave Preparedness: Children Vulnerability and Recovery", has looked into the possibility of Covid affecting children and the required strategies to deal with the pandemic. The recommendations made by the committee include "a holistic home care mode, immediate increase in paediatric medical capacities and prioritising mental health issues among children". It has mooted structuring of Covid wards in a way that allow kids' attendants to safely stay with them through their recovery.'

The public campaign to tackle Covid-19 in Mumbai, meanwhile, took concrete shape. The unique tactic Mumbai enjoyed was the ability to deploy hoardings. Mumbai has 1,150 public hoardings. This is far more than any other Indian city. Mumbai is a linear city with north-south and east-west road connectivity. Hoardings and billboards have high traffic movement and visibility.

'The city's hoarding owners were in continuous touch with me,' recalls Chahal. 'Following the national lockdown, they had poor business. I spoke to them on 8 September. This massive campaign was designed to begin on 15 September. They had been asking for some relief as even in September 2020, over 7 months after the pandemic arrived in India, there was hardly any outdoor advertising business. Corporates were simply not doing any marketing in light of reduced traffic on the roads. I asked the group of hoarding owners during our meeting: in these 1,150 hoardings that you control in the city, how many do you think you can use commercially between 15 September and 15 November? There were around 20 members of the hoardings association at the meeting with me. They said not more than 20 per cent of the hoardings will be sold commercially. Around 80 per cent will remain unused between 15 September and 15 November due to reduced economic activity.

'I told them that since these approximately 800 hoardings, nearly 80 per cent of the total, would lie vacant, it wouldn't matter much if they were with them or with the MCGM. I had not yet disclosed to them that our mask campaign and several other campaign initiatives were coming up shortly. They allowed us to take over around 800 unused hoardings totally free of charge. I said they could pick the marketable 20 per cent among the 1,150 hoardings they required commercially. The MCGM would not seek to use those. We have a separate department which handles the hoarding licence policy. Each hoarding is licenced. A deputy commissioner is in charge of this.

'We have a GPS behind every hoarding and a licence for each hoarding which is renewed on 31 March every year. So each hoarding is accounted for; no one can put up a hoarding in Mumbai without the MCGM's licence. The hoardings association wanted their licence fees to be made zero from April to September 2020 due to the fall in business. The MCGM collects ₹10 crore every month from them in licence fees. So it would be a loss of ₹60 crore for them if they paid the licence fee for those 6 months without any business. We assured them that the MCGM would work out a relief package for them.

'We eventually agreed to give them 4 months relief in licence fees from April to July 2020 because it would be unfair to ask them to pay a licence fee when business was shut. In return, we asked them to give us those 800 currently unused hoardings free of cost for 2 months from 15 September to 15 November for our Covid-19 campaign. Their licence fees from April to July would be written off. The hoarding owners would not incur any loss as the number of hoardings they gave us were anyway lying idle. They were happy with this arrangement and immediately signed the agreement.'

The Covid-19 educational campaign appeared in three languages: 60 per cent of it was in Marathi, 20 per cent in English and 20 per cent in Hindi. 'The hoardings had to be kept simple as people don't read in a moving car or bus,' points out Chahal. 'By 16 September we had put up 800 hoardings in Mumbai. Next, we printed pamphlets. This campaign made a big difference. People across the city, in high-rise apartments and tenements, became aware of the importance of Covid-appropriate behaviour. In the deadly second wave of the pandemic in the summer of 2021, Mumbai would otherwise have experienced 25,000 daily cases like Delhi did.'

Besides 800 hoardings, the MCGM placed stickers and posters on 3,500 BEST buses with the slogan 'No Mask No Entry'. It plastered gas/petrol stations with the same slogan. Shops too had 'No Mask No Entry' posters placed at key counters. 'The campaign is ongoing and has now become permanent,' says Chahal. 'All MCGM employees were involved in distributing campaign stickers to malls, shops and the cloth market. Around 45 lakh stickers were pasted in government and private offices, malls, small stand-alone shops, taxis, buses, public transport and trains—we had put up the stickers everywhere. Hoardings eventually had to go as they had a time limitation. But all the stickers remain. Simultaneouly, we started fining citizens ₹200 if they were found without a mask in public. A free mask was also handed over to penalised citizens. Mumbai has fined 3.7 million people found not wearing a mask in public.'

Chahal adds grimly, 'The virus is still among us.'

In the first Covid-19 wave through 2020, cases had emerged initially in Kerala and Maharashtra. They then spread to the rest of the country. The same pattern was replicated in the second wave in 2021. Kerala and Maharashtra accounted for over half the country's cases. In Maharashtra, Mumbai proved an exception. 'As the second, highly infectious wave began,' Chahal recounts, 'we launched yet another campaign on 24 February 2021 called "I Am Responsible". Besides this, "My Mask My Safety" was the slogan in all three languages on different hoardings. We wanted every citizen to be responsible and show responsible behaviour to get over this pandemic. It started with "My Family My Responsibility", then "Maha Kasam" for the sake of Maharashtra state, and then "I Am Responsible". No other city in the country has carried out this kind of concentrated campaign in a continous series, one after the other.'

When cases again began to climb steeply in April 2021, the Maharashtra government doubled down on its campaign 'Me Jababdar' ('I am Responsible'). Says Chahal: 'For this campaign too, we put up hoardings, but now we paid for them. On 27 November 2020, we had started the "Maha Kasam" campaign. M stands for mask, A is for *antar*, meaning distance in Marathi, and H for *hath*, which means hand. Maha Kasam means big promise. These hoardings appeared all over the city with three children emphasising the importance of masks, physical distancing and sanitisers. Children are a potentially vulnerable demographic in the next wave and this campaign resonated with them.'

Though cases and deaths had stabilised, a door-to-door campaign was now planned. 'We created 15,000 teams,' reveals Chahal. 'Each team had 3 to 4 people: a health worker, a *nagarsevak* or local political representative, an *anganwadi* worker and an NGO worker.

These 15,000 teams covered 1 lakh families per day at the rate of 6 families per team. The teams were first given a manual which had detailed instructions for individuals, families, societies, workplaces and shopping markets. On the back of the manual were the 24 ward war room phone numbers. These went to every city home. Today, nobody can say that they do not have our ward war room contact numbers.

'When the MCGM team came to your home, they first gave you the manual, spent 2-3 minutes explaining what was written in it, then checked the temperature and oxygen levels of all family members. In case your oxygen levels were low, they informed the relevant ward and you were admitted to a Covid Care Centre or a Covid hospital. If there was any comorbid person in the household who was bedridden, then a comorbid list was given to the health department with instructions to visit these patients at home and if needed shift them to a nearby health facility. The health workers recorded a photo with each family. We currently have 35 lakh photographs with us. The Tata Institute of Social Sciences (TISS) has done a third-party audit. We gave them our full data. The audit report analyses the impact of our mass campaign in Mumbai.'

The Epidemic Diseases Act of 1897 gives the MCGM wide powers to conduct health campaigns. 'We had told our teams that from the richest of the rich to the most powerful of politicians, everybody must be covered,' says Chahal. 'That is how, whether it was Amitabh Bachchan, Mukesh Ambani or Uddhav Thackeray, every single person was visited at their homes by one of our 15,000 teams. People like actors Aamir Khan and Anil Kapoor made videos thanking the MCGM for checking on them at their homes during the pandemic. The teams visited all homes, including those in the slums.

'The campaign covered almost one lakh families per day. We had to visit 35 lakh homes (two visits to each home) in 2 months. We devised a reporting format in 24 wards. The reports came to me on a Google sheet showing how many homes were visited that day. Every evening, a format was uploaded. The format had a large number of indicators, almost 20 items. For example: one, how many families has the team visited; two, how many hoardings have been put up; three, how many bus stops have been covered; four, how many manuals have been distributed out of the 45 lakh that were printed, and so on. We also used the electronic media through paid advertisements as well as FM radio and other media to emphasise the importance of the campaign and ensure Covid-appropriate behaviour on a long-term basis. This campaign will continue till the end of the pandemic and beyond.'

Chahal says that out of the 35.1 lakh families under the MCGM's jurisdiction, the civic body's 15,000 teams actually visited 34.99 lakh families. 'By doing so, even the common man believes that the civic body is looking after us,' says Chahal. 'Unfortunately, what happened is that the UK strain, later named Alpha by the WHO, became rampant in India after February 2021. It had first appeared in Britain in September 2020. At the time they said it was highly infectious but not lethal. As I mentioned earlier, when the Union government alerted us on 21 November 2020 about the presence of this UK Alpha mutant, we had acted swiftly. From the next day, 22 November we had imposed a complete 7-day total quarantine for passengers arriving at Mumbai airport from every country in Europe and the Middle East. Unfortunately, no other international airport in India—Delhi, Bengaluru, Hyderabad, Kolkata and Chennai—did the same. Mumbai was the only city to do this at the MCGM's behest. Any passenger from Europe, the Middle East, South Africa and Brazil was taken from the Mumbai airport to a hotel room and quarantined for 7 days. On the seventh day, we tested them.'

How did the Alpha variant, mutating to the Delta variant, spread through Mumbai and Maharashtra and trigger the second wave across the country in the summer of 2021? Chahal explains: 'Chandigarh has international flights to and from Dubai. Delhi has a lot of international flights to and from all major cities. These Indian cities did nothing at all. Passengers were arriving unchecked in India. It was only in February 2021 that Delhi decreed that UK passengers coming to India would be quarantined.

'It did not help much as people from these infected countries had already taken flights from Delhi and Bengaluru to Mumbai. In Punjab, 81 per cent of patients were found to be infected with the Alpha variant. It was highly infectious and spread rapidly. That is why the number of cases went up so quickly. We had written to the Union government that all airports should follow Mumbai's 7-day quarantine rule for all arriving passengers from 22 November. Nothing happened.'

EIGHT

POST-PANDEMIC INFRASTRUCTURE SURGE

Mumbai wrestled with several options to control the highly infectious Covid-19 pandemic. The question though remained: are lockdowns, partial or total, useful or necessary whenever there is a spike in cases? Sydney and Melbourne went into lockdown for months in 2021 despite small, localised outbreaks. Outbreaks in Southeast Asia sent several cities into lockdowns too as Covid-19 continued to rage through late 2021 despite vaccination rollouts. Britain chose a different path. It opened up the country on 19 July 2021 following a successful vaccination rollout. Maskless crowds returned to sports and entertainment arenas. So, however, did cases and fatalities—the highest in Western Europe. Omicron fuelled the panic.

Will India and Mumbai suffer a similar fate if there is a fresh wave or an intra-wave spike when they open up fully?

'In a pandemic whether you need curbs, restrictions, or a lockdown depends primarily on specific factors,' explains Chahal. 'When a city runs out of healthcare infrastructure, whether you get 100 patients in a day or 10,000 in a day is immaterial. The question is: if a city can handle 10,000 cases in a day and for every patient there is a bed waiting, then even if there are 10,000 cases there is no need for a total lockdown. The prime minister too, has acknowledged this. In a small town there could be just 100 cases but 50 cases don't get beds. A lockdown is dependent on your healthcare infrastructure and your capability to handle the pandemic surge.'

The Mumbai Model to combat Covid-19 was praised globally. But it took enormous effort to make it work, especially during the ferocious second wave.

Ripsa Chakraborty[38] described the cliff edge on which Mumbai walked during the pandemic:

> 'In April 2021, when the second wave of the pandemic was at its peak, the country's financial city recorded more than 10,000 daily cases thrice. The MCGM has garnered praise from across the nation. The Supreme Court not only applauded the management of medical oxygen supply in Mumbai, but also recommended that the Delhi government replicate the Mumbai Model to fight the pandemic. "When the first pandemic curve flattened post-November 2020, we used some Covid-19 beds for patients with non-Covid infections," said Suresh Kakani, additional municipal commissioner, health. "As soon as the number started soaring again, we upgraded our facilities. Initially, we had a limited number of ICU beds which were increased within a fortnight. Almost 40 per cent of Covid Care Centres (CCC) were activated and the remaining were kept on standby. If we are expecting (future waves) it is imperative that we vaccinate as many people as possible. Along with the elderly, we also want to inoculate the younger population who possibly would be more affected in the next wave"'.

Chahal notes that on 10 February, when the second wave ravaged

[38]*Hindustan Times*, 26 May 2021.

the city, Mumbai had 12,000 DCHC and DCH beds on the MCGM's live dashboard. 'Last year when we increased our capacities, we had constructed the hardware for 22,300 beds in Mumbai without touching the existing non-Covid beds,' Chahal points out. 'Our capacities were increased through Jumbos and by putting additional beds in Covid sections of various hospitals. When cases started increasing, we started increasing the number of beds from the 12,000 beds that we had on 10 February, 2021 to 14,752 beds on 3 April 2021 as the surge gathered force, and to over 30,000 beds in June 2021 even as the wave abated. Today, the situation is vastly different—and stable. The dashboard shows only beds which are operationalised where all the staff is available and where the patient can just go and start treatment. This dashboard is monitored by 240 doctors who are stationed in the 24 wards. They can't book a bed which is not operationalised.'

By June 2021, it was decided to reserve the 11 Jumbos for Covid-19 patients and increase the number of beds for non-Covid patients in private and public hospitals where Covid bed occupancy had declined with the cases abating. The MCGM meanwhile prepared paediatric wards in all its Jumbo hospitals to take care of children vulnerable to succeeding waves or surges. City paediatricians have been trained according to the ICMR guidelines and the protocol set by the Covid task force.

The policy followed by the Maharashtra government to contain the highly contagious Delta-led second wave had centred around imposing a gradually intensifying lockdown in April-July 2021 before equally phased out relaxations in August-December 2021 to minimise the impact on the economy, jobs, students and migrant workers who suffered enormously in the first total national lockdown. In a pandemic, experts say, a small number of infected people can be superspreaders. One person can infect up to 200 people. At the peak of the second wave in May 2021, there were relatively few cases in Mumbai's slums. Dharavi showed an uptick (which declined to near-zero in mid-July), but a greater number of cases emerged from high-rise buildings. Affluent citizens had abandoned Covid-appropriate behaviour during the lull in January 2021 when cases across the city dropped dramatically. They paid the price as several hundred buildings in upmarket locations were sealed. It took months for the crisis to pass.

The 'R' value fell below 1 in June 2021, lowering chances of infectivity, before rising again marginally as the city opened up during the festival season in late 2021. The MCGM imposed Section 144 during the Ganesh Chaturthi festival, prohibiting the assembly of more than 5 people. Caution remained the watchword through Diwali and Christmas as Omicron cases rose.

According to domain experts, total lockdowns are counter-productive beyond a point. Three experts explained why lockdowns should be temporary and localised. These domain professionals bring significant experience and knowledge to the debate. Maru Subramani is former CTO of Global Scholar and an engineer at Microsoft Research. He is currently a researcher at Bhaktivedanta Vidhyapitha Research Center, Mumbai. M.S. Seshadri is former professor of medicine and clinical endocrinology at Christian Medical College, Vellore, and currently medical director, Thirumalai Mission Hospital, Ranipet. T. Jacob John is former professor of clinical virology, Christian Medical College, Vellore.

In a joint article,[39] they explained the complex nature of lockdowns:

> 'What's the best time to impose a lockdown? Data from different parts of the second Covid wave can help governments make better decisions in future. A lockdown has serious adverse effects on the social, economic and psychological well-being of people, so it should be applied only when essential, and called off as soon as it starts doing more harm than good.

[39] *Times of India*, 14 June 2021.

The purpose of a lockdown is to retard the speed of virus transmission. Therefore, it is most beneficial when transmission speed or momentum is accelerating, but the benefit-risk ratio reverses as the momentum begins to decelerate. The epidemic curve ascends when one infected person infects more than one susceptible person—that's when infection's effective reproduction number (Re) >1. The curve descends when one infected person infects less than one other person (Re <1).

'Lockdowns during the rapid phase of increasing transmission help to minimise the Re and reduce it to less than 1. When Re<1, the epidemic will continue to decline naturally. In this situation, harm due to a lockdown outweighs any benefit. Even after unlocking, all states must focus on applying a "social vaccine" besides the "biological vaccine". States with declining mortality and surplus essential items like oxygen concentrators and drugs should consider sharing these with needy neighbours.

'A social vaccine consists of information-education-communication plus behaviour-change education for Covid-appropriate mask-wearing and physical distancing—which can be relaxed to arm's length if all are wearing masks—avoiding crowds, good ventilation of all closed environments, cough-sneeze etiquette and hand hygiene. Actually, a lockdown should be resorted to only after the full use of the social vaccine. The value of social vaccine was a lesson India had taught the world during the HIV-AIDS pandemic. We failed to learn from history and suffered the consequences during the Covid-19 pandemic. If we use both social and biological vaccines effectively and achieve wide coverage quickly, we can prevent a potential future wave.'

Looking ahead, Chahal is bullish about transforming Mumbai's civic infrastructure even as he keeps a watchful eye on the still mutating Covid-19 variants amidst the vaccination rollout for children. The long-lived pandemic ironically allowed Mumbai's ambitious infrastructure projects to move ahead rapidly despite a temporary shortage of workers. 'Due to the various lockdowns, there was free movement on vacant roads of raw materials required for heavy construction work,' points out Chahal. 'Several projects have taken off during the pandemic. For example, the Mumbai Coastal Road project is being undertaken by the MCGM. It will reduce travel time, decongest roads, reduce noise pollution levels, improve public transport by providing bus lanes, and generate additional green spaces. The coastal road starts from south Mumbai near the Princess Street flyover at Marine Drive. We began work on it in October 2018, but got stuck due to litigation in the Bombay High Court and then in the Supreme Court. On 9 June 2020, the chief justice of India heard a PIL and finally cleared the project.'

Chahal believes the coastal road will transform Mumbai: 'This mega project has three interchanges: the Amarsons interchange which has four exit arms and four entry arms, the Haji Ali interchange with eight arms, one arm each going to Peddar Road, Tardeo Road, Mahalaxmi Road, Worli Seaface, etc and the Worli interchange with six arms. The length of these interchanges together is 15.66 kilometres. Besides these, there are two tunnels, one northbound and one southbound. The length is 2.072 kilometres per tunnel. Each tunnel will have four lanes. The unique feature of the coastal road project is that it involves the largest diameter tunnel excavation ever done by a tunnel boring machine in India. The machine is 12.19 metres in diameter—the largest diameter machine ever used in the country. It has a monopile foundation system, again a first in India. The project will reduce travel time from Marine Drive in south Mumbai to Bandra in north Mumbai, past the Bandra-Worli Sea Link, by almost 70 per cent.

'Fuel consumption of vehicles will reduce by an estimated 30 per cent. The coastal road will allow signal-less travel, so there will also be a reduction in noise pollution. Additional green space of 70 hectares is being created along the coastal road, accessible to the public. The entire green belt of 175 acres is abutting the original coastline and the coastal road is 150-500 metres beyond that. We have created a large parking space under the green belt. There will be dedicated bus lanes so people can get off a bus and walk into the garden. These are public gardens that the 16 million citizens of Greater Mumbai will have total access to.

'The actual expenditure on the project is ₹12,777 crore. There is zero loan and zero grant from the central government. The money is from the MCGM's reserves. It is a unique project where a municipal organization is building a coastal road worth almost $2 billion with zero financial assistance from anybody else. Tenders were issued by the MCGM. We issued the work orders. No funding from the government of India or the government of Maharashtra was taken. We took no bank loans. Most, if not all, road projects or metros are built with loans. The coastal road is a loan-free project. The project will be completed by November 2023. Building a 14-lane coastal road with two tunnels, in the heart of Mumbai city, completing it on time: one can imagine the speed at which the work is going on. We have been advised by expert groups, with absolute seriousness, to invite the National Geographic and Discovery Channel to portray this as a mega urban project meriting international recognition.'

Chahal is equally optimistic about upgrading post-pandemic Mumbai's access to clean water: 'Since 2011, Mumbai was planning to covert its sewage water into potable water. Roughly 24 million litres per day of sewage water can currently be converted into potable water. To increase the amount of water supply in Mumbai due to an increase in population, Mumbai would have to build two new irrigation/drinking water dams, Gargai and Pinjal. These will be somewhere off Thane in a rural area. We already have five water dams to augment supplies.

'To build drinking water dams, more than 4,50,000 trees would have to be cut. Because of this, the proposal is stuck with the environment department. Next, we will have to build 120 kilometres of pipelines to get this water. Experts advise that we should convert sewage water into potable water instead. The technology is expensive, but in the longer run we will save 4,50,000 trees and save on building infrastructure as well. There are more than 1,000 sewage treatment plants in action in the world today. This is a ₹20,000-crore project. We propose to build 7 STPs (Sewage Treatment Plants). One would be located at Worli with a capacity of 500 million litres per day (mld). A second STP will be built at Bandra (360 mld), a third at Dharavi (418 mld), a fourth at Versova (180 mld), a fifth at Malad (454 mld), a sixth at Bhandup (215 mld) and a seventh at Ghatkopar (337 mld). Their combined capacity would be around 2,464 mld. The idea of cutting 4,50,000 trees to build Gargai and Pinjal dams is shelved now.

'For this ambitious project, tendering was attempted between 2011 and 2019, but due to various reasons the tenders would periodically get cancelled. Vested interests would try to get the terms and conditions changed, try to fit in local players, bring in their own contractors. This would lead to controversy and the controversy would lead to cancellation of the tender. The latest such incident happened in July 2020. I made a commitment to the Maharashtra government that we must get the best possible quality as per the accepted terms and conditions. We shall not change a single para, full stop or comma once we finalise the terms and conditions through the experts—come what may. There will not be any interference at all.

'We did a lot of homework and hired one of the world's best consultants. There are only four technology providers who are considered the best in the world. One is a company in France, another in the US, a third in Singapore and a fourth in Israel. These are the leading companies which have done research and which possess top-of-the-line technology. Earlier tenders had called for the EPC contractor to construct the plant. Once they won the bid, the EPC contractor would find the technology partner. But there could be a compromise on the technology as the contractor might choose a local vendor and compromise on quality.

'So we made two major changes in the tenders which were getting cancelled time and again. Between 2012 and 2020, all governments tried but all failed due to a lot of interference. Vested interests continued to intrude. If they did not get the bid, they started complaining. Ultimately, the project got ambushed. We therefore decided on a protocol. Number one, top tech players can bid but no one shall get more than one project. We made that a precondition. Earlier one firm could get all the projects. Number two, the technology partner has to be one of these four top global STP firms that we had identified. We then gave freedom to these select technology partners to sign MOUs with any number of local vendors. They could all bid. Whoever gets selected is assured of the best global STP technology. This was a landmark decision which killed the repeated decade-long cancellation of tenders.'

Chahal encountered opposition from entrenched lobbies but held firm. He says: 'We told everybody that they cannot question our credibility or say that we are dictating or limiting the competition. At the end of the day, our satisfaction lies in the fact that all 7 STP projects are being built under the technology of top global tech partners. They are the best in the world in their field. For example, at Singapore's Changi airport, you get bottled water that is 100 per cent recycled water from a sewage treatment plant. It is the most sought after bottled drinking water in Singapore.

'When this project takes off, it will substantially increase Mumbai's potable water capacity. It will suffice for Mumbai till 2060. People initially resisted this project, but eventually they fell into line. STP technology providers based in India too, strongly opposed the project. But we put our foot down, and hats off to the CM. He said there will be zero compromise on quality, so except these few global STP companies no one else was entertained. For once there was strong political leadership. The small players kept up their interference but to no avail. The full project cost of ₹20,000 crore is being funded from our own resources. The 7 STP potable water projects will take 4-5 years to complete but they are on track and will benefit Mumbai tremendously.

'Mumbai is the financial capital of the country, a global city. We have lagged behind in sewage treatment. When I went to Adelaide in Australia, which has a population of only one million, I saw how people are converting sewage water into drinking water. Many cities in the world are using recycled water. The way the water crisis is looming over Mumbai, water is an increasingly precious commodity. This project is excellent because we are using recycled water which we can recycle again and again. We don't need to cut down lakhs of trees, there's no need to maintain dams, no need to maintain pipelines, no need to spend thousands of crores on building new dams.'

In yet another concerted bid to modernise Mumbai's post-pandemic infrastructure, the MCGM plans to construct a hydro-electric and a solar plant at the Vaitarna dam, becoming one of the rare municipalities to build a hydro/solar power project and generate its own electricity. Explains Chahal: 'We decided to build this 20 MW hydro-electric power plant. I had served as an officer in the irrigation department and had a fair idea about floating solar panels to generate solar power. So we planned a hybrid project of 80 MW floating solar panels and 20 MW hydro-electric power. Since I had worked as irrigation secretary for 4 years, I knew that 24 per cent of the water in an irrigation dam can evaporate in one year. Evaporation is high at 40 degrees celsius summer temperatures. Over one-fourth of dam water evaporates in a few months. Experts confirm that when floating solar panels are placed to cover the dam it reduces evaporation. Less evaporation means more water to use, plus you get 80 MW of power.

'This is a public-private partnership (PPP) project. We discussed how to get top engineers to run the solar power plant. We needed new recruits, new manpower. We therefore decided to float a bid for solar panels where the bidder has to invest in the 20 MW power plant and quote a price at which they will sell power to us. We will sign a power agreement with whoever gives us the cheapest power rate per unit. Private players have to contribute the total investment. We will put the power on the national grid so that it can be used anywhere in the country. We have got clearances for this ₹536-crore project. The bidder has to pay ₹536 crore and quote a power unit rate for 25 years at around ₹4.75 per kilowatt hour. Presently, thermal power is available at ₹5 per unit. We will buy power from the bidder at ₹4.75 per unit and save on thermal power generation. We will be saving an estimated ₹25 crore per year. The MCGM today buys power from the Adanis or the Tatas, so this will be our net saving per year. After 25 years the entire project will be handed over to us. We would then become owners of the power plant.'

Meanwhile, the ₹6,600-crore Mulund-Goregaon link tunnel is a key infrastructure project set to be completed as Mumbai comes to terms with the new normal in life and work. Residents of Thane and Mulund currently travel from the eastern suburbs to the northern suburbs like Goregaon, Dhaisar and Borivili, undergoing a harrowing 2-hour drive. East-west connectivity in Mumbai is not as good as south-east and north-south connectivity. The Goregaon-Mulund connectivity project was planned way back in 2005. It is finally getting off the ground now.

'The project has three phases,' says Chahal. 'The most important aspect in this Goregaon-Mulund link road is that we have to cut through Sanjay Gandhi National Park. This national park is a reserved forest. We have to go 92 metres under the national park, building two tunnels, each with a length of 4.7 kilometres. The total project cost is ₹6,600 crore. When this complex project is completed in 2026, vehicles can go from Goregaon to Mulund in just 15 minutes, a journey that today takes over 2 hours. The entire project cost of ₹6,600 crore is again being borne from the MCGM's reserves. None of these projects are dependent on loans or on the support of the Union government or the Maharashtra government. It is our own initiative and our own money.'

As he continues to marshal the vaccination drive, Chahal regards adversity as an opportunity to further upgrade Mumbai's civic development. 'I have been hearing talk about desalination plants in Mumbai for years,' he says. 'Since Mumbai has a long coastline, a desalination plant is an ideal solution to Mumbai's water problems. A feasibility study was being conducted by an Israeli company which is a world leader in desalination plants. There are several parametres which are very important in building a desalination plant. First, the quality of sea water should be very good. The eastern coast in Mumbai is more polluted than the western coast because of harbours and ships. Second, the location of the desalination plant should have enough natural bodies to store water there. To store water in artificial ponds and tanks is very expensive. Third, mangroves should not be present in the desalination area.

'The consultants took a year to work on various suburban areas like Versova, Bandra, Manori, Wadala and Madh island. After all these on-the-spot studies, they finally recommended Manori, which is between Versova and Madh island. At Manori, they have recommended a 200 mld desalination plant, as natural water bodies are present there. Water is also cleanest there. This 200 mld plant will cost us ₹1,800 crore. But it is worth it. The alternative of building a dam like Gargi, cutting 4,50,000 trees and constructing a 100-kilometre pipeline, is not viable. It is so much better to have a desalination plant of 200

Social Media, especially Twitter and Facebook, was full of praise for Iqbal Singh Chahal's proactive work as Commissioner of the MCGM during the darkest days of the Covid-19 pandemic.

Featured on these pages is a sample of tweets – ranging from government leaders to Bollywood stars – recognising the work done by Chahal and his 'army' of 1,08,000 MCGM staff.

At the peak of his career, Chahal possibly became the first IAS officer to trend on Twitter by his name.

Amitabh Bachchan
@SrBachchan

T 3895 - Mumbai fights .. may it inspire others too ..” prayers 🙏

YouTube

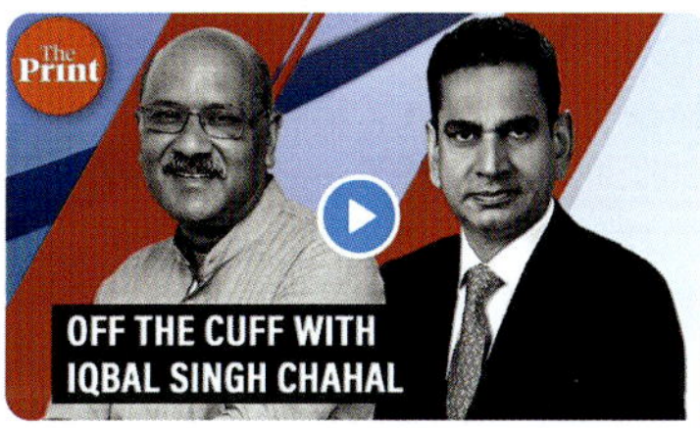

Off The Cuff with Iqbal Singh Chahal
#ThePrintOTCBrihanmumbai Municipal Commissioner Iqbal Singh Chahal was our guest at ThePrint's latest Off The Cuff. In a conversation with Editor-in-Chief Sh...

Sudhir Suryawanshi
@ss_suryawanshi

The Supreme Court praises the @mybmc for its work containing the virus & bringing down positively rate. It says BMC has done the remarkable work & asked Delhi govt to look at BMC model & follow some good things to control the situation in Delhi. @NewIndianXpress @Sunday_Standard

1:49 PM · 05 May 21 · Twitter for Android

Rajdeep Sardesai
@sardesairajdeep

I haven't seen a more focussed bureaucrat than @IqbalSinghChah2 in this Covid fight. Mumbai owes him a huge debt although fight has some way to go. Helps to be a marathon runner in real life! Hope Delhi too has a single point fully empowered local authority. 🙏

anand mahindra
@anandmahindra

The Municipal Corporation of Mumbai was proactive in managing Covid 19 at the outset, a bit complacent in between, when there seemed to be a lull in cases, but has quickly played catch-up. Today, its dashboard is a template for other cities. 👏👏👏(1/2)

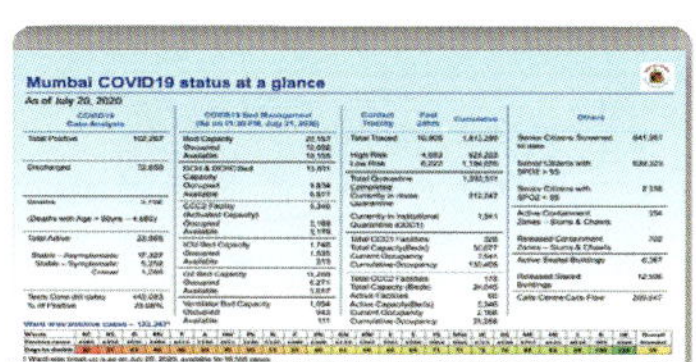

10:49 AM · 22 Jul 20 · Twitter for iPad

anand mahindra @anandmahindra

More good news from Mumbai that people—around the world—should see. A report from @mybmc Commissioner Iqbal Singh Chahal. Evidence that crisis management skills are alive & well. A 👍 for the preparation for any 3rd wave.

In Mumbai, despite high inflow of Covid patients, we have more than 4090 vacant beds in 172 Covid hospitals on MCGM's online integrated real time bed allotment dashboard available on my cell phone. We have increased the number of beds from 12000 to almost 22000 in the last 6 weeks, adding 1500 more beds at NESCO Goregaon this week.

Even the number of ICUs have been increased from 1500 to almost 2800 now.
We increased the number of ambulances from 300 to 700 in the last 4 weeks.

We are amicably resolving oxygen issues for the city of Mumbai. We have 2 Municipal auditors posted in each of the major private hospital in Mumbai to ensure that patients are charged at Government rates only, i.e. Rs. 4000/-per oxygen bed, Rs. 7500/-per ICU bed and Rs. 9000/-per ventilator bed. Mumbai is the only city in India where all positive reports of the patients are received by MCGM in single line list from all testing labs at midnight and thousands of patients are informed early morning through MCGMs 24 ward war rooms managed by more than 700 doctors in 3 shifts.

requiring hospital beds to assess their medical condition and then allot eligible category of bed in these 172 hospitals at their residence.

I wish to humbly submit that, in the second wave which started on 10th of February 2021, the total number of new cumulative positive cases have been 3.09 Lakhs & total number of cumulative deaths have been 1319.

The mortality rate for the second wave has been 0.4% and this is lowest anywhere in the world.

Besides,7 functional Jumbo field hospitals in Mumbai comprising of more than 9000 Covid beds, MCGM has already started building 4 new Jumbo field hospitals at Malad, Kanjur Marg, Sion and Worli Race Course comprising of 5000 beds and 800 ICUs which will be ready in next 4 weeks so that we are well prepared for the 3rd wave in Mumbai which may or may not hit us in the future.

Team MCGM will leave no stone unturned to effectively

12:09 PM · 26 Apr 21 · Twitter for iPhone

Manjinder Singh Sirsa @mssirsa

Hats off to the vision, passion and humility of @mybmc Commissioner @IqbalSinghChah2 who is Mumbai's COVID hero and India's brand ambassador to the world

He credits this success as Waheguru's blessing

India cannot be written off until we have visionary IAS officers like him

The Economist London quotes him as the man whose Data-driven planning made saved Mumbai from Covid wave. Washington Post, Singapore CNBC, Reuters & top media groups of every country has highlighted his role in saving Mumbai. The Chahal Model stands tall with statistics as incredulous as Mumbai's death rate just 0.6% (Lowest in the World)

Even Supreme Court praised BMC for handling Covid-19 and asked Delhi Govt

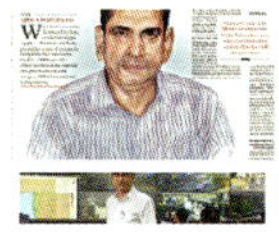

REPUBLICWORLD.COM LIVE TV

Mumbai floats global tender to acquire 1 crore COVID-19 vaccines: BMC Commissioner Chahal

The Municipal Corporation of Greater Mumbai has issued a global bid today to acquire 1 crore COVID-19 vaccines to vaccinate citizens against COVID in Mumbai

Written by Pritesh Kamath

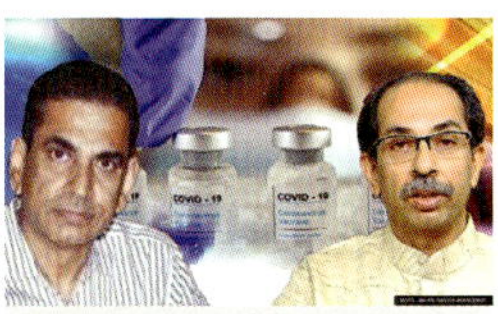

IMAGE: PTI/AP

Kiran Mazumdar-Shaw @kiranshaw

I just studied the Maharashtra and BMC model of decentralised Covid management n super impressed with it's uniquely thought out processes Kudos to @OfficeofUT n @mybmc n its dynamic Iqbal Singh Chahal 👏👏👏 The whole country should follow these COVID beating methods

9:01 AM · 10 May 21 · Twitter for iPhone

Kiran Mazumdar-Shaw @kiranshaw

Mumbai Model Gets World Attention | IAS Iqbal Chahal on beating COVID | ... youtu.be/cO48XBronMg via @YouTube
Decisive leadership based on data n decentralisation is the way forward. I wish the country would emulate Chahal's logic of cost of vaccination Vs cost of treatment

YouTube

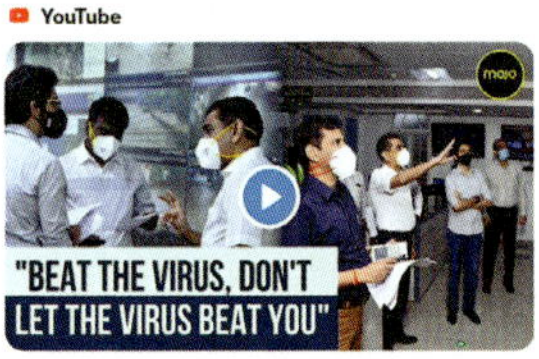

Mumbai Model Gets World Attention |

Amitabh Kant @amitabhk87

Centralized bed allotment, anticipating oxygen storage facilities, common allotment of beds even in pvt hospitals, dashboards for monitoring , war rooms for patient follow up. Inspirational Mumbai model of Covid Mngmnt . Congrats @mybmc Commissioner Chahal & his Gr8 team.

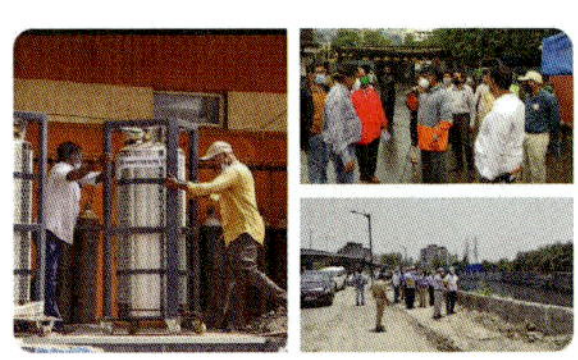

12:01 AM · 10 May 21 · Twitter for iPhone

Javed Akhtar
@Javedakhtarjadu

I believe others need to learn a lesson or two from the government of Maharashtra and Bombay Municipal corporation that are fighting with the menace of COVID with with tremendous competence .

11:46 PM · 08 May 21 · Twitter for iPhone

Hardeep Singh Puri
@HardeepSPuri

The way BMC Commissioner Iqbal Singh Chahal has blunted the impact of Covid in Mumbai to a very large extent shows how a right approach & judicious use of resources including oxygen (not press conferences over it) is all it takes to turn the tide.

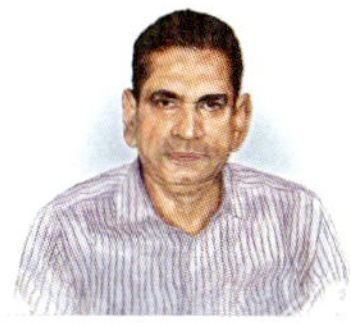

indianexpress.com
Iqbal Singh Chahal: If Mumbai has 6-7% positivity rate, why should we suffer a nationa...

Jyotiraditya M. Scindia
@JM_Scindia

Shri Iqbal Singh Chahal has done a spectacular job of managing the crisis in Mumbai. In this interview, he recounts how GOI's swift action on his SOS call for oxygen helped save lives. A fine example of cooperative federalism!

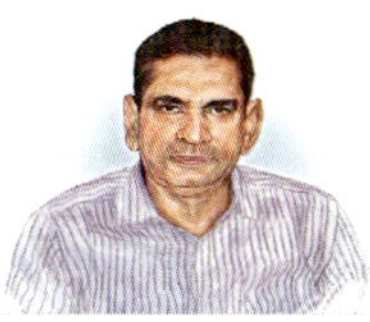

indianexpress.com
Iqbal Singh Chahal: If Mumbai has 6-7% positivity rate, why should we suffer a nationa...

5:42 PM · 10 May 21 · Twitter for iPhone

Sucheta Dalal
@suchetadalal

Mumbaikars... please note. Thanks to the guts shown by municipal commissioner @IqbalSinghChah2 and @mybmc there is plenty of #Remdesvir available at all civic hospitals. The facilities are also safe. Please consider opting for it in emergencies and save your loved ones!🙏

5:57 PM · 19 Apr 21 · TweetDeck

Bar & Bench
@barandbench

Justice Chandrachud: If the health secretary of Delhi Govt and centre has a meeting with Iqbal Singh Chahal of Mumbai Municipal Corporation and draw from experience and tell us how you plan to create storage tanks and install it for Delhi.

1:35 PM · 05 May 21 · Twitter Web App

Kailash Kher
@Kailashkher

महाराष्ट्र मुम्बई में स्थिति सुधर रही है जिसका श्रेय हमारे योग्य एवं कुशाग्र अधिकारी ब्रहनमुंबई महानगर पालिका आयुक्त @IqbalSinghChah2 के कुशल नेतृत्व तथा उनकी समर्पित टोली को.जो रात दिन अपनी निष्ठा से इस चुनौती का सामना कर रहे लोगों का जीवन बचा रहे. @mybmc #IndiaFightsCorona

Indian
@Arpita16967690

Replying to @IqbalSinghChah2

U r d only govt official in my entire lifetime whose autograph I would want to have & click a pic with. And there are many like me thx to d the way u handled Covid.I remember ur interviews & best thing was how u used to explain the prep work backed by no's.U rock MR Commissioner!

9:23 AM · 20 Jul 21 · Twitter for iPhone

Ronnie Screwvala
@RonnieScrewvala

Mumbai's Covid Fight Model has been internationally acclaimed and there's one man to be credited for it- @IqbalSinghChah2 Commissioner @mybmc. Much deserved #MumbaiRatnaAward. Congratulations and thank you for all the efforts in the battle against #Covid19

Pic: @IndianExpress

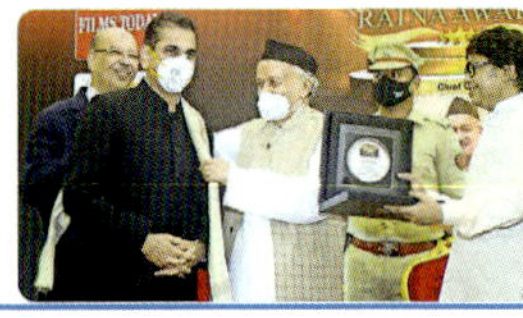

Bloomberg
@business

Mumbai has reported a quarter of the Covid deaths in New Delhi, since the new wave began on March 1.

Iqbal Singh Chahal, Mumbai's municipal commissioner, tells @BloombergTV how the world's second-densest city managed its virus crisis trib.al/XppGVUK

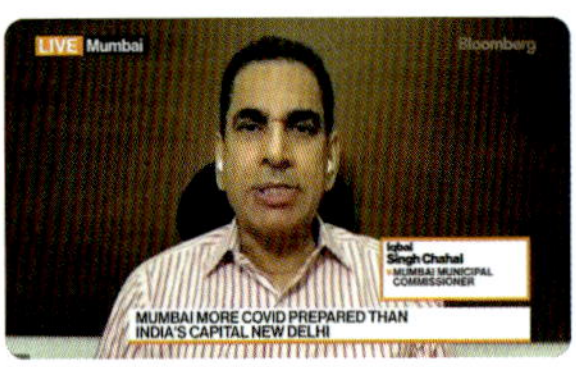

19.6K views

sohit mishra
@sohitmishra99

लोग 1375 किलोमीटर का सफर एम्बुलेंस से तय कर मुंबई आ रहे हैं केवल बेड और बेहतर अस्पताल सुविधा के लिए.. हाल ही में सुप्रीम कोर्ट ने भी बीएमसी की तारीफ की.. यह मुंबई के लिए ज़रूर गर्व की बात है,लेकिन दूसरे इलाकों के हालात कितने खराब हैं आप उसका अंदाज़ा इसी से लगा सकते हैं...

Translated from Hindi by Google

People are coming to Mumbai after traveling 1375 km by ambulance only for beds and better hospital facility.. Recently Supreme Court also praised BMC.. It is definitely a matter of pride for Mumbai, but for other areas You can get an idea of how bad the situation is...

U.S. Consulate Mumbai
@USAndMumbai

.@mybmc Commissioner Iqbal Singh Chahal joined #CGRanz today for a tour of our operations, including #DostiHouse and our consular team hard at work processing student visas. As part of the Mumbai's community, we appreciate all of BMC's support!

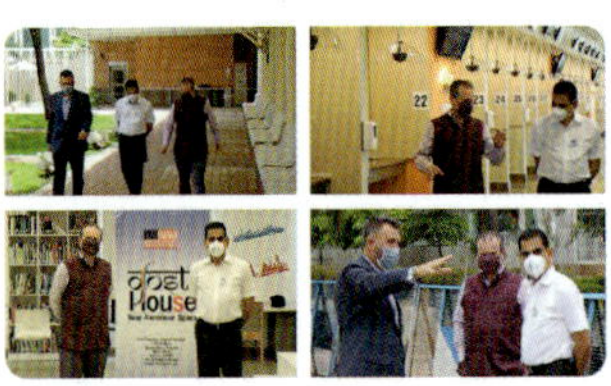

4:28 PM · 23 Jun 21 · Twitter Web App

Anant Goenka
@anantgoenka

One of mom's colleagues called me to help his pregnant 32 yr-old get an ICU. I didn't make any special "calls"..only followed the advertised war room numbers... it took time but was surprised by how efficient @mybmc was in communicating and resolving. Patient is doing well now.

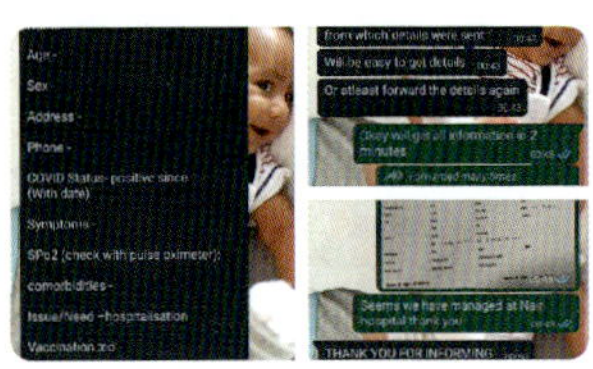

7:18 PM · 30 Apr 21 · Twitter for Android

Chahal used WhatsApp to innovative effect during the Covid-19 pandemic. He created over 30 groups comprising more than 6,500 eminent people – political leaders, diplomats, Indian and foreign journalists in print, electronic and online media, IAS officers, IPS officers, senior doctors and judges.

The impact was immediate. Information flowed in real time in both directions – from Chahal to his audience and to Chahal from his audience. Inaccurate news was swiftly countered. Doubts were cleared. The Mumbai Model was decoded.

On these pages are a sample of the messages received by the MCGM Commissioner during the Covid-19 pandemic.

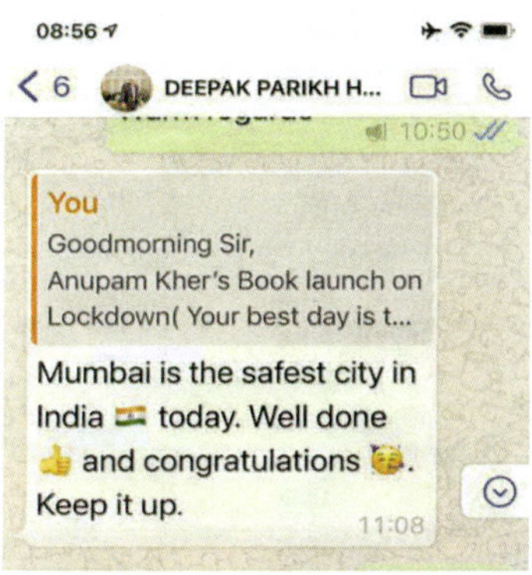

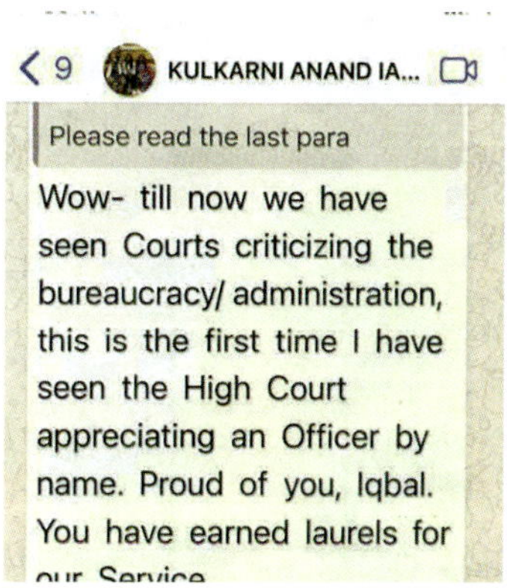

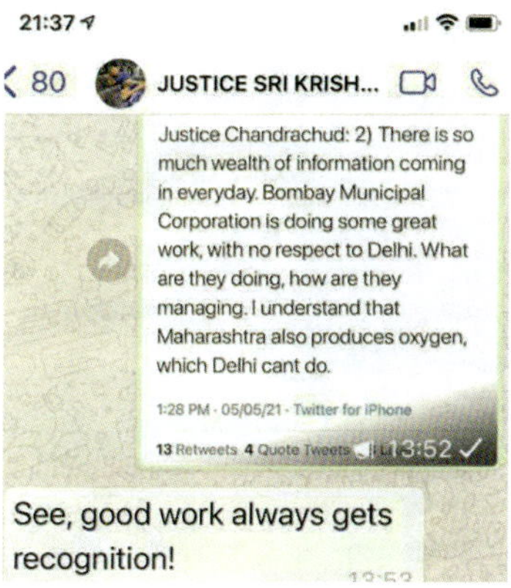
21:37
80
JUSTICE SRI KRISH...
Justice Chandrachud: 2) There is so
much wealth of information coming
in everyday. Bombay Municipal
Corporation is doing some great
work, with no respect to Delhi. What
are they doing, how are they
managing. I understand that
Maharashtra also produces oxygen,
which Delhi cant do.
1:28 PM · 05/05/21 · Twitter for iPhone
13 Retweets 4 Quote Tweets
13:52
See, good work always gets
recognition!

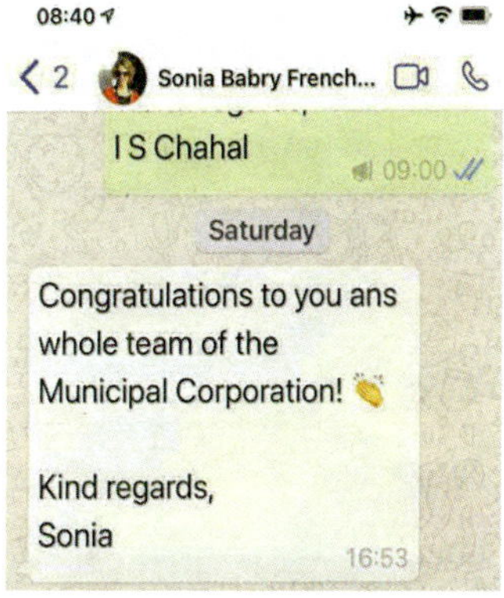
08:40
2
Sonia Babry French...
I S Chahal
09:00
Saturday
Congratulations to you ans
whole team of the
Municipal Corporation!
Kind regards,
Sonia
16:53

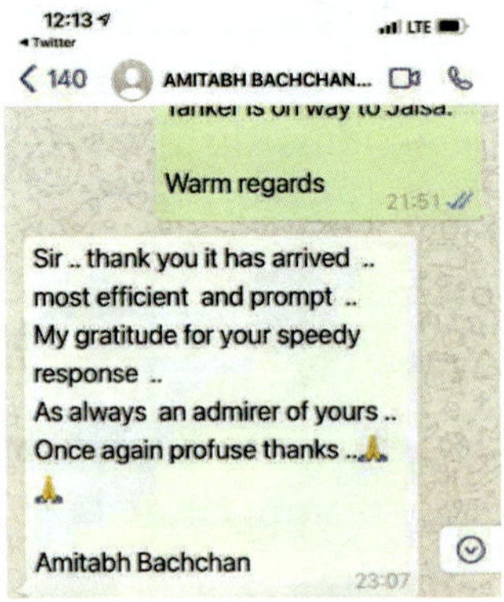

12:13
Twitter
140 AMITABH BACHCHAN...
Warm regards
21:51
Sir .. thank you it has arrived ..
most efficient and prompt ..
My gratitude for your speedy response ..
As always an admirer of yours ..
Once again profuse thanks ..🙏
🙏
Amitabh Bachchan
23:07

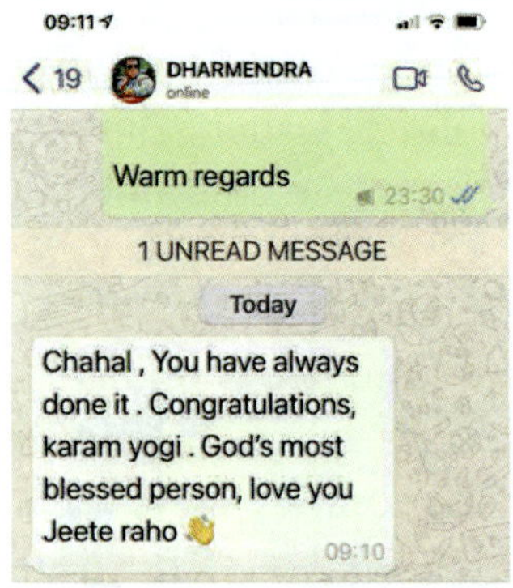

09:11
19 DHARMENDRA
online
Warm regards
23:30
1 UNREAD MESSAGE
Today
Chahal , You have always done it . Congratulations, karam yogi . God's most blessed person, love you
Jeete raho 👋
09:10

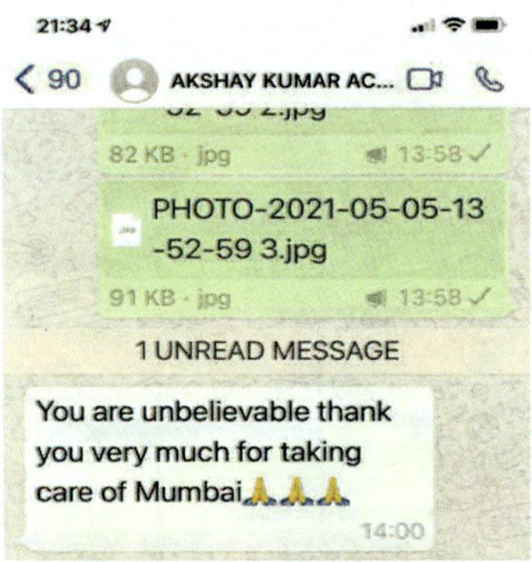

21:34
90 AKSHAY KUMAR AC...
82 KB · jpg 13:58
PHOTO-2021-05-05-13-52-59 3.jpg
91 KB · jpg 13:58
1 UNREAD MESSAGE
You are unbelievable thank you very much for taking care of Mumbai🙏🙏🙏
14:00

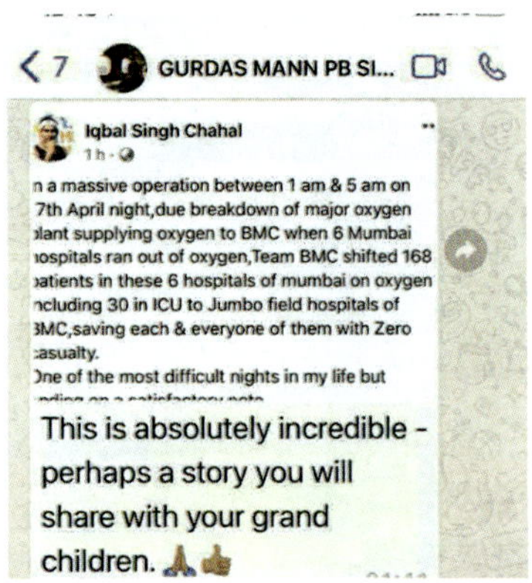

7 GURDAS MANN PB SI...
Iqbal Singh Chahal
1h
n a massive operation between 1 am & 5 am on 7th April night,due breakdown of major oxygen plant supplying oxygen to BMC when 6 Mumbai hospitals ran out of oxygen,Team BMC shifted 168 patients in these 6 hospitals of mumbai on oxygen including 30 in ICU to Jumbo field hospitals of BMC,saving each & everyone of them with Zero casualty.
One of the most difficult nights in my life but
This is absolutely incredible - perhaps a story you will share with your grand children. 🙏👍

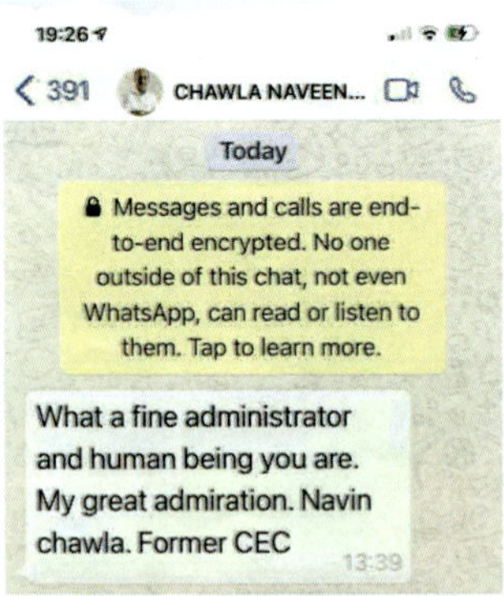

19:26
391 CHAWLA NAVEEN...
Today
Messages and calls are end-to-end encrypted. No one outside of this chat, not even WhatsApp, can read or listen to them. Tap to learn more.
What a fine administrator and human being you are. My great admiration. Navin chawla. Former CEC
13:39

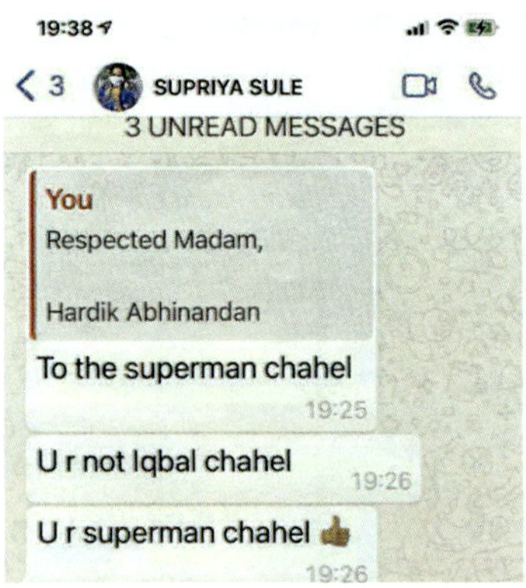

19:38
3 SUPRIYA SULE
3 UNREAD MESSAGES
You
Respected Madam,
Hardik Abhinandan
To the superman chahel
19:25
U r not Iqbal chahel
19:26
U r superman chahel 👍
19:26

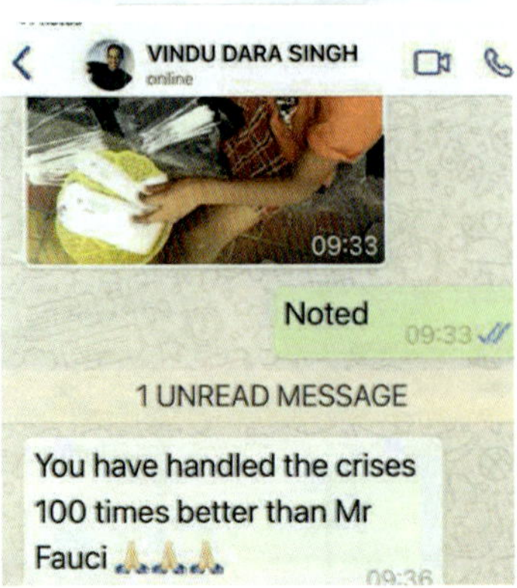

VINDU DARA SINGH
online
09:33
Noted
09:33
1 UNREAD MESSAGE
You have handled the crises 100 times better than Mr Fauci 🙏🙏🙏

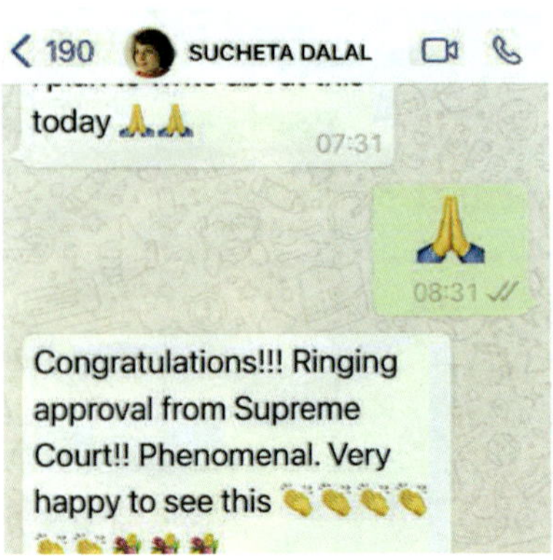

190 SUCHETA DALAL
today 🙏🙏
07:31
🙏
08:31
Congratulations!!! Ringing approval from Supreme Court!! Phenomenal. Very happy to see this 👏👏👏👏

10:33
B B TANDON IAS RET...
online

Warm regards 08:15

1 UNREAD MESSAGE

Superb and superb, saw the entire interview. State/ Nation is blessed to have officers like u.
Allow me to share with a wider audience.
Proud of u. Regards 10:32

18:22
MAGO ARUN IAS
online

1 UNREAD MESSAGE

Congratulations Chahal ji for a great job in an extremely difficult and challenging situation. I am sure Maharashtra cadre will be proud of your efforts.
Excellent interview.
Warm regards
Arun K Mago 16:59

12:09
ANU MALIK SINGER

Dearest dearest respected IS Chahal saheb - congratulations -

You sir deserve every bit of this honour as you have been at the forefront in this fight against COVID & have managed to control the 1st & 2nd wave effectively and have succeeded in controlling its spread-

I salute you and your entire team at Bmc-

Personally also very very proud of you IS Chahal saheb
Warmest regards
Anu malik 00:07

You sir are truly a true Ratna of mumbai 00:07

08:51
GAIKWAD RATNAK...

On Christmas, Mumbai`s Dharavi records zero coronavirus cases , India New...
Unbelievable 👍🙏 08:03

Mr Chahal, you successfully tackled what can be called just a miracle! Everyone was so worried about Dharavi 08:03

09:14
MULLICK SUMIT IAS CS

BMC
Mumbai 08:25

It's really very commendable. Dharavi will become a case study in universities around the world.
And you will go down in history 👏👏 08:48

🙏 09:14

17:15
JOSEPH JHONNY

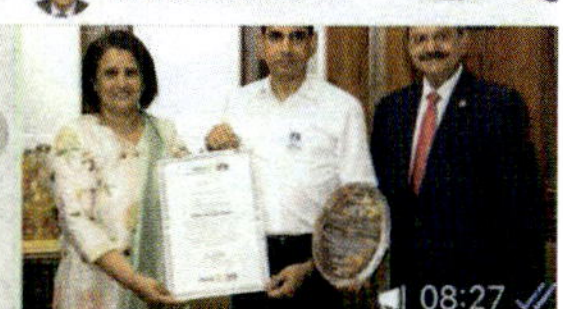
08:27

A great feather in your crowning cap of unparalleled achievements !
Remarkable. Hearty congratulations ! 08:50

KULKARNI ANAND IA...
online

Warm regards 08:19

You
Respected Sir,

Pls spare time to watch my inte...

A role model for other IAS officers in the country. Efficient handling, to say the least. Keep the flag flying high, Iqbal 08:54

10:41
APURVA CHANDRA IAS
online

COVID RESPONSE MODE in detail.

Warm regards 08:22

Hats off Iqbal. It is exhilarating to listen how you managed Covid in Mumbai. Should be made compulsory listening for all administrators and Doctors 👍👌👍 08:48

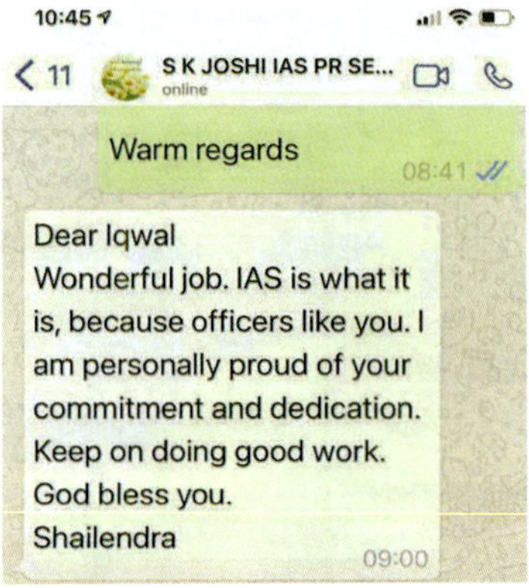
10:45
11
S K JOSHI IAS PR SE...
online
Warm regards
08:41
Dear Iqwal
Wonderful job. IAS is what it is, because officers like you. I am personally proud of your commitment and dedication.
Keep on doing good work.
God bless you.
Shailendra
09:00

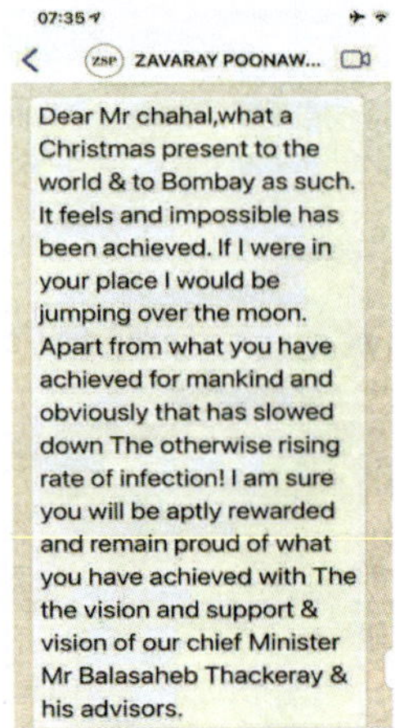
07:35
ZAVARAY POONAW...
Dear Mr chahal,what a Christmas present to the world & to Bombay as such. It feels and impossible has been achieved. If I were in your place I would be jumping over the moon.
Apart from what you have achieved for mankind and obviously that has slowed down The otherwise rising rate of infection! I am sure you will be aptly rewarded and remain proud of what you have achieved with The the vision and support & vision of our chief Minister Mr Balasaheb Thackeray & his advisors.

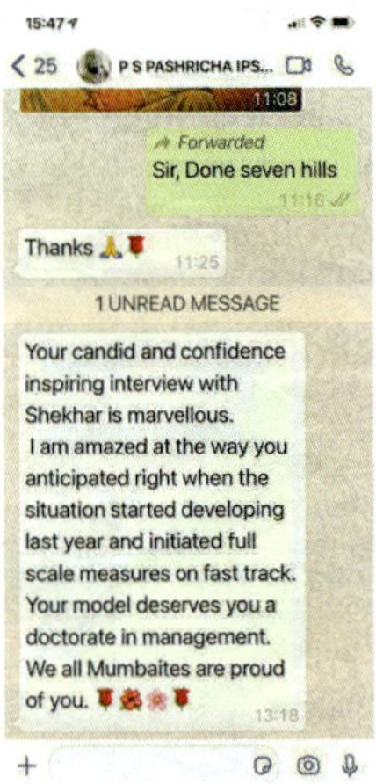
15:47
25
P S PASHRICHA IPS...
11:08
Forwarded
Sir, Done seven hills
11:16
Thanks 🙏🌹
11:25
1 UNREAD MESSAGE
Your candid and confidence inspiring interview with Shekhar is marvellous.
I am amazed at the way you anticipated right when the situation started developing last year and initiated full scale measures on fast track.
Your model deserves you a doctorate in management.
We all Mumbaites are proud of you. 🌹🌺🌸🌹
13:18

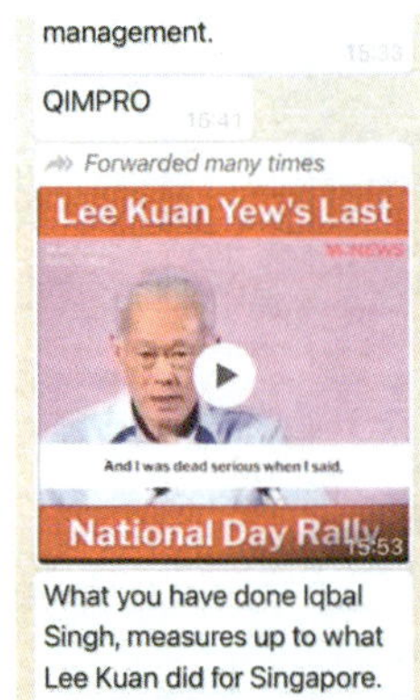
management.
QIMPRO
Forwarded many times
Lee Kuan Yew's Last
And I was dead serious when I said,
National Day Rally
15:53
What you have done Iqbal Singh, measures up to what Lee Kuan did for Singapore.

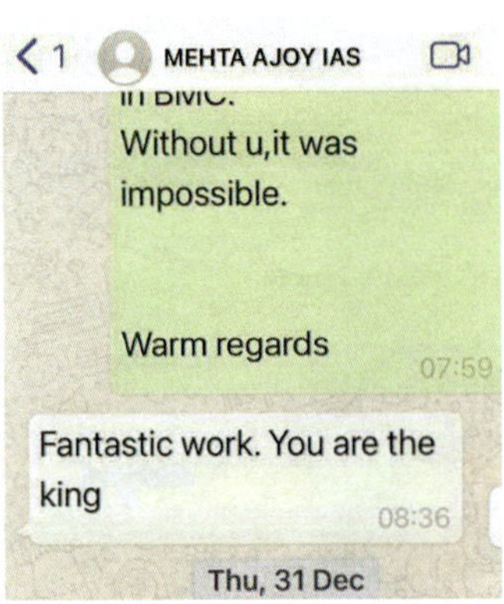
1
MEHTA AJOY IAS
in BMC.
Without u,it was impossible.
Warm regards
07:59
Fantastic work. You are the king
08:36
Thu, 31 Dec

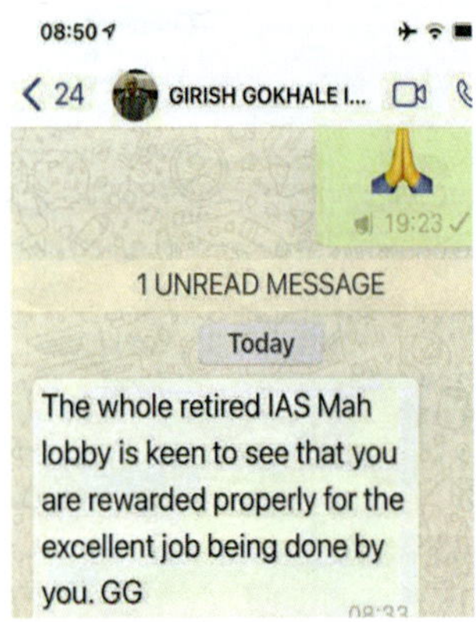
08:50
24
GIRISH GOKHALE I...
🙏
19:23
1 UNREAD MESSAGE
Today
The whole retired IAS Mah lobby is keen to see that you are rewarded properly for the excellent job being done by you. GG

mld without cutting a single tree. There are 1,015 desalination plants functioning in the world presently. There's a 1,000 mld plant in Saudi Arabia. Sydney has a 500 mld plant. There is enough technology available in the world. This will be a permanent asset for Mumbai after the pandemic is over.'

Other critical issues, however, remain unresolved. Housing for the civic body's staff has been a perennial problem for the MCGM. 'An important welfare project for which we have issued work orders,' says Chahal, 'involves building homes for MCGM workers. Many municipal workers live in very dilapidated quarters. Some were built before independence. Most are on prime land. Real estate developers tried to convince office bearers of the MCGM to undertake a redevelopment project. Certain flats would be given free of cost to the civic body. On the remaining land, the developers would build luxury flats and sell them in the market. In this tug of war, with real estate developers entering this project, there was zero headway.

'When I came in as commissioner, we decided to remove all the developers. For specific sites, we proposed to directly issue a tender, appoint a contractor to build the housing project for us and use its full potential. How much would it cost us? There was tremendous resistance to this proposal from certain lobbies. But I had the support of the CM. I explained to him that our corporation has 29,618 sweepers. These new houses are basically meant for them. They can get good accommodation provided we spend some funds and do it ourselves rather than rely on developers. The project is now underway at 10 locations with good quality contractors. It is a clean deal where you get a contractor, pay him and get the work done, no land dispute, no land sharing, no sharing of roads, no redevelopment sharing, no questions that somebody has got less or more area, or someone has got a larger share in the land. It is very clear cut and transparent, like building your own house, finding a contractor and paying him. This project will benefit the poorer workers of the MCGM.'

Singed by the second Covid-19 wave in mid-2021, the MCGM has also begun upgrading several hospitals in Mumbai and building new ones. Says Chahal: 'We are building a brand new Kasturba Hospital and Sion Hospital. We have 5 major MCGM hospitals—KEM, Sion, Cooper, Nair and 7 Hills—and 13 peripheral hospitals. This year we are spending ₹5,000 crore on health upgradation. We have started work on a new medical college in Vile Parle, the Balasaheb Thackeray Medical College, at a cost of ₹290 crore. We will construct a new building for the medical college. We are redeveloping and constructing a new building for Bhagvati Hospital in Borivili on a budget of ₹486 crore. These are all contractual works. We also have a new construction, Govandi Hospital, at ₹501 crore, a ground-plus-eight-storey structure. We are building MP Agarwal Hospital in Mulund for ₹457 crore and Bhabha Hospital in Bandra for ₹287 crore. We are constructing two basement, ground and two-storey buildings with 496 beds. All this medical infrastructure entails a total expenditure of ₹5,000 crore and will fully prepare us in the event of future waves of the Covid-19 pandemic.'

How will the MCGM fund its ambitious infrastructure and healthcare projects? 'The first mental block,' Chahal says, 'was whether the corporation's ₹70,000 crore reserves should be kept as they are or be pumped back for the welfare of citizens? That was the turning point. We took the decision to utilise our reserves rather than borrow.'

Chahal returns to his theme: Mumbai needs a single planning authority. He elaborates: 'Worldwide, cities have a single planning authority. It is the planning authority which plans the development of the city for the next 10, 20, 30 years. For example, the MCGM has created a development plan for 2034. Every inch of land is reviewed in Mumbai and then planned: what should be the reservation here, what should be the activity there. The plot may be private or government.

We have to plan whether there will be a residential project here, or commercial, or hospital, or school, or garden, or road. If someone's private land is involved, that person will get compensation. If government land is involved, then work will proceed quickly.

'Mumbai, unfortunately, is a city with multiple planning authorities. For example, BKC is out of our jurisdiction. The MMRDA is BKC's planning authority. For slums, SRA is the planning authority. For 56 colonies in Mumbai, MHADA is the planning authority. The Mumbai Port Trust again is a separate planning authority. After setting aside all these, the MCGM is the planning authority for the rest of the city. My speech on this in the 2021-22 budget ruffled many feathers. I repeated the suggestion in a letter to the government. I said, in the interest of Mumbai, please abolish all the planning authorities and make MCGM the single planning authority. It means MMRDA, MHADA, Port Trust and SRA should all be removed as planning authorities. Today, the planning authority for Dharavi is SRA. So besides SRA, nobody can plan, issue a tender, invite a bidder, redevelop or construct anything there. Unless the MCGM is declared a planning authority there, except for supplying drinking water and electricity and managing sewage, we have no other role to play. Dharavi is prime land. It can be redeveloped into a modern colony. But we need the authority to do it.'

For the moment though, Chahal had more pressing worries: the Covid-19 pandemic had reached an inflection point in Mumbai. Or had it?

NINE

OXYGEN: BREATH OF LIFE

Unlike Delhi, where cases and fatalities kept rising in the last week of November and much of December 2020, Mumbai witnessed a continuous decline in cases and deaths. 'By mid-January 2021, our positivity had come down to 1.52 per cent,' says Chahal. 'We were getting only around 300 cases every day, at times just 270 or 280. At that time Dr Neelima, the dean of the NESCO Jumbo, which we believe is the largest field hospital anywhere in the world with 3,000 beds and 224 ICUs, met me. She said she had only 3 patients in the NESCO Jumbo for the 3,000 beds and no patients in the 224 ICUs. The Jumbo was fully staffed. The 224 ICUs were outsourced and we were paying 50 per cent minimum guarantee to our outsourced vendor. It would have been natural to ask: why not shift these 3 patients to another hospital? We had 184 hospitals on the dashboard. We could have closed this Jumbo. The Jumbo is where the National Exhibition Centre was. There was demand from the trustees to vacate the area. But I had a hunch that we were still not out of the woods. So I told the dean: let the Jumbo carry on. I told her to meet me a few months later and then we would take a call on what was to be done.

'My hunch proved right. Within 3 weeks, on 10 February 2021, the second wave started. Nobody had predicted it. In Mumbai, the fact that we did not allow the closure of the NESCO Jumbo shows that we knew a second wave could come and were prepared for it. We had 9,000-plus beds in the 7 Jumbos. Not a single bed was closed. We had only 250 to 300 patients being admitted every day at the end of January 2021. Still, not even one bed was reduced or even one Jumbo hospital closed.'

By now, the MCGM had allowed selective surgeries of non-Covid patients. Later, as the second wave swept through Mumbai, these were again halted. On 10 February, the city had 1,800 asymptomatic patients. There were 3,000 symptomatic patients from all over the Mumbai Metropolitan Region (MMR). 'From MMR, anyone is welcome to come directly and occupy a bed,' says Chahal. 'So from 14 April 2021, the graph went up steadily. On 14 April, we had 93,000 active cases. From 2,000 Covid-19 patients in February, the number shot up to 93,000 patients on 14 April.'

These numbers would continue to increase steadily every day. On 4 April, Mumbai recorded over 11,100 Covid-positive cases, the highest for the city in a single day during the second wave.

'The second wave created a lot of stress on our infrastructure because we were getting between 8,000 and 11,000 cases per day,' recalls Chahal. 'The only saving grace was that unlike how things were during the first wave, symptomatic and asymptomatic patients were now in the ratio of around 50-50 or at most 60 per cent symptomatic and 40 per cent asymptomatic. In contrast, during the first wave the ratio was 83 per cent symptomatic patients and 17 per cent asymptomatic. On 10 February 2021 the cumulative positive cases in Mumbai since the beginning of the pandemic in March 2020 was 3.13 lakh; on 31 May 2021, when the second wave began to ebb, the total cumulative cases were 7.06 lakh. Thus in the second wave, we recorded nearly 4 lakh positive cases in a short period of just over 3 months. But fortunately the mortality rate was just 0.8 per cent, as I said one of the lowest in any comparable city globally. When the first wave ended, Mumbai's mortality rate was 3.65 per cent. Bringing the mortality rate down to below one per cent in the second wave was a tremendous achievement. In contrast, the death rate across the entire country was much higher during the second wave than it was during the first wave. 'The main reason why we achieved significant success in lowering the mortality rate was the systems we had put in place. The Mumbai Model consists of 28 principal sub-models and almost all of them are now on autopilot. So when the second wave confronted us, the system kicked in automatically. Our ward war room concept, integrated dashboard with 186 public and private hospitals and real-time, integrated, single-point of allotment of hospital beds made us the one city in the world where the test report does not go from the testing lab to the patient directly. All the several lakh test reports done so far have gone through the MCGM to the patients. Although we started this practice on 8 June 2020, not even one other city in the world has emulated us. That is because it is a highly risky decision. Even if a single mistake happens that the report comes first to the MCGM and the patient dies, then the patient's relatives could sue us, stating that the patient died due to negligence and the unnecessary requirement that test reports come only through the MCGM.

'I am happy to say that there has been razor-sharp precision in the process. Till today in Mumbai, there is not a single complaint on record either in writing or in the media that a patient's report has gone missing. I had said on day one that everything should be put on software where there is no human intervention. In infotech, it is not possible that even one entry could go missing. This has proved to be right in all our test samples. But other cities have not taken this risk as they might be apprehensive that if some reports go missing, there could be a major crisis with a patient dying due to negligence on the part of the authorities and subsequent legal action. So this was a unique model created and successfully operated by us.'

With reports in the Indian and foreign media of bodies floating on the Ganga River in Uttar Pradesh and corpses buried in shallow watery graves going viral, attention turned to the shortage of crematoriums during the virulent second wave. Mumbai has 47 crematoriums with a capacity of 1,350 cremations per day. All the crematoriums are booked online. Against this total capacity of crematoriums, the single highest number of deaths in one day in Mumbai was 77.

Other cities were less fortunate. As the second wave gathered momentum, there were calls to reduce crowds at election rallies, especially in West Bengal. By April 2021, it was clear that the huge crowds the election campaign was drawing could be superspreaders. The spike in Covid-19 cases in West Bengal in May and June confirmed the critics' worst fears.

The Kumbh Mela in Uttarakhand, attended by millions of devotees, was another superspreader in the midst of the brutal second wave. It was eventually called off before its scheduled close in the face of mounting criticism, including from health experts in the Union government. Dr V.K. Paul, a member of Niti Aayog and the Covid task force, conceded: 'Standard operating procedures related to the coronavirus pandemic should have been followed in letter and spirit in the Kumbh Mela and rallies in states which went to the polls. We must bring the focus back on our behaviour. There is no place for creating crowds, there is no place for not wearing masks. That is the only way we can break the chain of transmission.'

In Mumbai, meanwhile, with hospital bed rates still capped, the availability and cost of life-saving medicines assumed serious proportions. All MCGM hospitals treat patients free of charge and most medicines are free as well. Says Chahal: 'However, I had several cases where a patient's relatives called me from various private hospitals and said that critical medicines were not available. I told one VIP patient that I cannot supply the required medicines from the MCGM's stock due to our protocol. But if he would like, I could send an ambulance to pick him up and admit him in a Jumbo hospital. If he wanted an oxygenated bed, or an ICU bed, we could provide it. Everything is free. So in the end, several dozen such influential patients came in. They moved mid-treatment from private hospitals to get free medication from the MCGM and we were able to save all of them. These patients were in private hospitals when they shifted. This was a unique situation—patients moving midway from private hospitals to government hospitals. It used to be unheard of.

'After this we created a "step-down" facility. HN Reliance Hospital, Hinduja Hospital and Bombay Hospital were overflowing with patients because, in the second wave, over 90 per cent of those affected were from affluent families. Only 10 per cent were from slums. Affluent patients preferred treatment at private hospitals. They did not mind paying. We were running short of beds. So we came up with a new idea. We linked Trident Hotel, Bandra, with HN Reliance Hospital; Bombay Hospital was linked with Intercontinental Hotel, Marine Drive, and Westin Hotel, Marine Lines. Two three-star hotels were linked to Surana Hospital and one hotel to Hinduja Hospital. All these hotels housed Covid-positive patients who did not require oxygen or ICUs. These patients had anyway been lying on normal Covid beds at HN Reliance and the other linked hospitals.

'Bombay Hospital assigned doctors and nurses to Intercontinental Hotel so that the patients housed there were taken care of. These hotels were empty during the second wave with thousands of Covid cases being recorded per day in Mumbai in April-May 2021. As and when a patient vacated a hospital oxygen bed, he or she was shifted to these linked hotels for recovery. The patients were moved to hotels as they were now out of danger or were asymptomatic. The hospital beds were needed for more seriously ill patients. In this way, we got hundreds of parallel beds with the step-down hotels initiative. As a step-down facility, they became extensions of the hospitals.'

In early April 2021, a review meeting was chaired by Maharashtra Chief Minister Uddhav Thackeray. Mumbai had 70,000 active Covid-19 patients at that time. The state had over 6 lakh active patients. These active patients were consuming 950 MT of oxygen every day. The total state-wide oxygen production capacity of Maharashtra was 1,200 MT of oxygen per day. Covid cases were rising. Within a week an oxygen crisis could well occur. Experts projected a daily requirement of 1,700 MT. Certain non-Covid patients under treatment for heart disease or cancer too, needed oxygen.

'In the first week of April 2021,' Chahal says, 'we banned elective non-Covid surgeries which used oxygen. But we still knew that we were staring at a great crisis of oxygen. Maharashtra, at that time, had the highest number of Covid cases in the country. Kerala would overtake us only later in the year. We were the first to ring alarm bells within the Union government, around 5 April, to allot us 500 MT of oxygen a day as we could not manufacture oxygen beyond our installed capacity.

'Neighbouring states had 5,000, 6,000 cases. We had more than 60,000 daily cases. Most oxygen production comes from steel plants which are under the union government's jurisdiction. The moment we took the matter up with the union government, it alloted us 500 MT of oxygen to be lifted by the state government partly from Haldia in West Bengal, partly from Vijaynagar in Bengaluru, partly from Visakhapatnam and partly from the Bhilai Steel Plant. I spoke to the chief minister. I said that to get oxygen from Haldia will take around 8 days. It is not a one-time affair. The tanker has to come every day. I said every state may have a Covid crisis and oxygen shortages. It will be difficult for tankers to move from one state to another.

'I sent four direct messages to the principal secretary to the prime minister, the cabinet secretary of India, the union home secretary, and the Union health secretary on the morning of 18 April 2021. It read: "Respected Sir, Good morning. I take this liberty to bring to your kind knowledge that 151 Covid hospitals under the MCGM, Mumbai, with more than 20,000 Covid-positive patients admitted presently are facing an acute problem of supply of oxygen. The situation is more or less the same in the rest of the state as well. Last night, 6 MCGM hospitals ran out of oxygen supply stocks. We had to launch a massive rescue operation at midnight to shift 168 Covid patients on oxygen, including 34 in the ICU, to our Jumbo field hospitals to save their lives. This went on till about 5.00 am. We have succeeded in saving all these precious lives. However, if our daily consumption of 250 MT of oxygen is not available, a major calamity and threat to the lives of the Covid patients cannot be ruled out. I am trying my best with the state government, but things look difficult. It is my humble request to help the MCGM in this time of crisis. The immediate solution could be to airlift vital oxygen supplies with the assistance of our defence forces. Kindly excuse me for sending you this message in such a grave crisis."'

Chahal got an immediate response: 'The cabinet secretary of India was sent this message at 11.32 am. Within 15 to 20 seconds, I received an incoming call from him. I explained the entire situation to him, but he said that they could not airlift oxygen because air force officials have explained its limitations. If a fully filled oxygen tanker is airlifted, it could explode in mid-air. Empty tankers can be airlifted, not full ones. Meanwhile, empty tankers were being airlifted, getting filled with oxygen and coming back by road or on a train. This is how the oxygen trains were started for the filled-up tankers.

'I requested the cabinet secretary to give us oxygen from Reliance Industries in Jamnagar. This is 16 hours away. It would be an overnight journey. I had already spoken to Reliance Industries Ltd. They were ready to supply the oxygen, provided the union government gave them permission to do so. It was very kind of the union government to grant us permission immediately. Mumbai was at the time using

235 MT of oxygen a day. The Supreme Court appreciated us for managing with just 235 MT of oxygen whereas Delhi was demanding 700 MT of oxygen a day.

'Our system of oxygen management has several key SOPs. The Supreme Court went over our entire management system. First, we created 5 emergency stock points with 50 MT storage capacity. Mumbai has 24 wards. For every ward we had one permanent tanker lying 24/7 ready to move in 5 minutes. We had cyclinders kept ready. Each centre was put under a deputy commissioner of the MCGM. We posted our officials at the Food and Drug Administration (FDA) office in BKC which was monitoring oxygen supplies for Maharashtra. If a hospital sent us a message that its oxygen stock was likely to be exhausted in another 2 hours time, in 3 minutes flat our tanker started moving. I had given strict instructions to all officers of the MCGM that if any of them gets an SOS call for oxygen, there will be a single point of forwarding: the call has to go to a ward officer as a single point of contact. The ward officer also has to forward the same SOS message to the deputy commissioner in charge, again a single point of contact. The deputy commissioner had the power to move the tanker.

'Each stock point centre had 8-10 MT of oxygen, 50 MT in all. The tanker moved and in 15 minutes the refilling of the oxygen cylinder at the hospital started. This was from emergency stocking. It was not difficult to spare this much oxygen—and even that can save precious lives. Without the emergency stocks, we cannot deliver oxygen at midnight if a patient's relative sends an SOS call. Key SOPs became a part of our oxygen management system:

1. Maintain saturation level of 94-95 or 98-99. No patient is going to die at 94-95 levels. This will save a significant amount of oxygen.
2. High-flow nasal oxygen is a guzzler and should be used only in rare cases.

3. Hospitals must audit oxygen stocks and usage—how many patients used how much oxygen last week and compare it to the present week.

'The Supreme Court appreciated our idea on saving oxygen. If the entire country followed these SOPs, there would be a 10 per cent saving on oxygen usage. Another key part of our SOPs was that when the oxygen tanker leaves, for example from the Jindal plant or the Reliance plant, we should be crystal clear whose tanker it is. I had told the state government very clearly that I would put armed people in the tanker when it leaves the plant unless the state government issues clear orders that the moment the tanker leaves the Jindal or Reliance plant it will come straight to the MCGM. This clarity was not there at many places in India. These SOPs led the Supreme Court to commend our efforts.'

Chahal cites the example of Hindu Mahasabha Hospital in suburban Ghatkopar which sent an SOS that its oxygen was finishing in the next 2 hours. It also informed one of the main Opposition leaders so that they could hold a press conference to embarrass the MCGM over shortage of oxygen stocks. Says Chahal: 'The moment I got the message, we swung into action. They did not know about my emergency stocking. In 11 minutes flat, the tanker reached Hindu Mahasabha Hospital. The Opposition leader who had scheduled the press conference came half an hour after the oxygen stocks had arrived. The press conference did not take place. I am grateful to the Supreme Court for encouraging us throughout the oxygen crisis.'

The possibility of a third wave—which the US and other countries were struck by in December 2021—worried the government and health authorities. Pressure Swing Adsorption (PSA) oxygen plants were set up all over India. Drug stocks were now plentiful. Vaccinations had proceeded well with vaccine hesitancy declining, though last-mile vaccination access for all adults and children remains a challenge.

Sandeep Poundrik, director-general of the Coalition for Disaster Resilient Infrastructure, put preparations for future Covid-19 surges in perspective[40]:

> 'While it may be difficult to predict the exact timing and magnitude of the next wave, it is possible to estimate its impact, based on the experience of the first two waves. These estimates can then form the foundation for preparing resilient health infrastructure to tackle a possible third wave.
>
> 'The Coalition for Disaster Resilient Infrastructure, launched by Prime Minister Narendra Modi in 2019, has published a working paper on this issue. The paper's estimates are based on the magnitude and timing of the second wave after scientific assessment, learnings from the experience of India and other countries, and advice from epidemiologists. It also recommends steps that the central and state governments must take to ensure adequate beds and oxygen for patients, if the next wave strikes. Assuming that the peaks at the state level will be at different times, the oxygen demand is expected to vary between 6,200 MT and 8,500 MT per day. However, in the unlikely situation of a peak beginning simultaneously in all states, the oxygen demand may shoot up to between 13,800 MT and 20,600 MT per day. Therefore, the authorities must prepare for the upper end of the spectrum.
>
> 'In the business-as-usual scenario, UP, Bihar and West Bengal are expected to require the most oxygen at 3,076, 1,818, and 1,344 MT per day, respectively, out of the total 16,387 MT average all-India requirement. Therefore installing

[40]*Hindustan Times*, 20 July 2021.

> Pressure Swing Adsorption oxygen-generating plants across India must take this into account rather than distributing them evenly across all states. Futher, states that do not have industrial oxygen production facilities must ramp up their oxygen capacity. Whether future waves occur or not, this is an opportunity for India to prepare the health infrastructure system for an efficient and quick response to such mega and unprecedented health challlenges.'

Additional Municipal Commissioner Suresh Kakani remains confident of tackling future waves of the pandemic. He said that the MCGM has an inventory of 30,000 hospital beds, including oxygen beds. He added[41]: 'We have scientifically worked to upgrade our oxygen facilities and ensure minimum wastage. As the first step, we switched from a cylinder-based system to a central oxygen supply as the former requires cylinders to be refilled every few hours. At the end of the second wave, we started upgrading to the central oxygen system.'

Mumbai's oxygen management protocol became a key element in the city's battle against the pandemic. Recalls Chahal: 'There were 83 deaths in Goa over four different incidents due to a shortage of oxygen in hospitals. I received a message early in the morning on 5 May 2021 from the health secretary of Goa, Puneet Goel, that he wanted to talk to me. It was around 8-8.30 am when I called him. He said Prime Minister Narendra Modi had called the chief minister of Goa and instructed that we must talk to Chahal on oxygen management. I spoke to Goa's health secretary for half an hour and told him about our SOPs, our systems. The population of Goa is only 16 lakh. It has around 25 hospitals. But subsequently, 83 people died from lack

[2]*The Times of India*, 20 August 2021.

of oxygen. There clearly was mismanagement. Systems have to be created and made to work on autopilot when you have a pandemic on a large scale.

'During the second wave, these autopilot systems really helped us. We must salute all our private sector hospitals. Although they had taken a financial hit due to the pricecap we placed on various hospital charges, they continued with the same tempo, the same level of co-operation. The pandemic will go away in a few months, but the hospitals' reputation has skyrocketed. Several global Indian CEOs flew into Mumbai in private air ambulances from Dubai and elsewhere to seek Covid treatment in the city's excellent private hospitals. One family—husband, wife and child—who became Covid-positive, couldn't get a hospital bed in Gurugram. They hired an ambulance for ₹1,10,000 and drove for 2 days from Gurugram to St. George Hospital in Mumbai. They got a bed, were admitted and in 5-6 days discharged in good health. There are countless other examples. A senior correspondent, Krishna Kumar with the *Economic Times*, Mumbai, was in a village beyond Chennai. He became Covid-positive and took an ambulance to Mumbai with his wife. It was a 1,700-kilometre drive. He was admitted to 7 Hills Hospital, and he is well today. We have treated Covid-19 patients from Srinagar, Lucknow and several other cities.

'That is the kind of trust we have built up. In Mumbai, name one VIP, journalist, retired IAS officer, sitting judge or an influential person, name one who has died from Covid-19 because of non-availability of either oxygen or a hospital bed. There has not been a single day when there was no bed available in Mumbai. At the peak of the second wave on 14 April, we had 3,600 vacant beds.'

Mumbai's obvious challenge now is taking care of children below the age of 18—both in terms of the vaccination rollout and paediatric facilities. There are clear sensitivities involved. Chahal says, 'If a one-year old child is Covid-symptomatic, then the mother has to accompany the child, the mother has to feed the child, so it cannot be in an open space ward. Privacy has to be provided. But what do we do in Jumbos where there are long halls? In the first week of May 2021, when we decided to build four new Jumbos, we made arrangements for paediatric rooms. The new Malad Jumbo has 2,165 beds and several hundred cubicles as well as 250 ICUs. We did a sero survey of children in the age group of 12 to 18 as preparation for the paediatric wave. We found very encouraging results: 51.5 per cent children have immunity. In the age group of 10-14 years, 54 per cent have immunity. These figures reassure us that the paediatric wave will get blunted. Furthermore, in the fifth sero survey conducted in the area under the MCGM's jurisdiction, antibodies were found in 90.26 per cent of the people who were fully or partially vaccinated. In unvaccinated citizens, 79.86 per cent were found to have antibodies.

'Besides creating 1,700 cubicles for mother-and-child, we have also built paediatric ICUs and paediatric ventilators. We have created a task force of paediatric doctors. These doctors hold physical meetings every Saturday and Sunday at ward offices with the general physicians of that area. They groom them for paediatric care, how to handle young symptomatic and asymptomatic patients. They have been given the task of creating a patient treatment protocol for both symptomatic and asymptomatic children.

'Till recently, we had 11 operational Jumbos—BKC 1, BKC 2, NESCO, Worli Dome, Dhaisar Naka, Mulund Naka, Richardson Crudas, Kanjurmarg, Sion, Malad and Worli Race Course. These 11 Jumbo hospitals have 11 in house oxygen plants and 15,200 beds, 70 per cent of which are oxygenated. We won't need to import oxygen in a future crisis. In 5 traditional MCGM hospitals, we have created captive oxygen plants with corporate funding. Many private hospitals have also put up their own oxygen plants. So our external requirement for oxygen will come down. Oxygen should not be an issue for Mumbai in the next wave.

'We have outsourced management of these four new Jumbos too. They are fully equipped with ICUs, ventilators, oxygen, suction pipes, monitors, beds, etc. Except for the staff, from ward boy to medicos, the Jumbos are handled by professionals from private hospitals. Several corporate houses have pitched in with generous donations. The total funds the MCGM received in the first wave has been surpassed multiple times by the money it has received through CSR (Corporate Social Responsibility) donations in subsequent waves of the pandemic.

'I always say that history is going to judge us by mortality, not by the number of Covid-positive cases. I got a very nice message from Ajit Seth, who was union cabinet secretary from 2011 to 2015. He wrote that he and his colleagues were very proud of what we were doing.' *The Economist,* frequently and obsessively critical of India, was meanwhile moved enough to publish an article titled: 'How the city stayed a step ahead of the coronavirus', adding that 'there is no equivalent of Mr Chahal in Delhi.'

Much of Chahal's success in fighting the Covid-19 pandemic can be attributed to his willingness to take calculated risks. From creating 24 ward war rooms to building Jumbo field hospitals, he has shown an ability to take calculated risks, something which is rare in a senior IAS officer. Mentoring fledgling IAS officers, Chahal addressed 182 probationers at the IAS academy in Mussoorie for more than 2 hours in the summer of 2021. He recalls: 'When they were just finishing their training I was invited to address them. I told them that unless they have a risk appetite they will not succeed in public service.

'In public service, most of the decision-making is in grey areas. Every decision would be scrutinised by all the stakeholders. The second advice I gave them is to be optimistic. If they are optimistic, they will solve more problems of the people. The third and last point I made was that if they meet 10 people every day, their intention should be to help all 10, whoever may come in front of them, whether it's a chairman, a deputy commissioner, an assistant a commissioner, commoner, etc. They must immediately put themselves in the person's shoes and gauge how important their work is. The person you are meeting has come with a lot of hope, don't brush him aside. When you leave your home in the morning for office, you may end up meeting 10 to 50 people. To do everyone's work is just not possible. It is very difficult to deliver all the time, but with positive intent you may be able to help 4-5 people among the many you meet every day. But if you are not optimistic and positive, and if you don't put yourself in their shoes, you may not be able to help even one person.'

Chahal also shared with his audience that during the second wave, he had received nearly 200 WhatsApp messages from lower income groups, and from people living in the slums in particular, seeking urgent hospitalisation for their loved ones. Says Chahal: 'Our strike rate was 100 per cent. We created a system where we would directly allot a bed/ambulance in a few minutes to these unknown and vulnerable citizens. All these unknown WhatsApp messages from these unknown people still exist in my mobile phone. Many of then would send a message of thanks after 15-20-25 days, when the admitted person was discharged, to express their gratitude. Some messages even thanked me for my timely help even though ironically and sadly, the admitted patient passed away after 2-3 weeks. Nothing though can be more satisfying than saving a human life.'

Chahal adds reflectively: 'It was a good address to the IAS probationers. Out of 182 IAS probationers, 100-plus subsequently sent me messages and became my friends on social media. They told me that during the 2 years of their training, they had serious, informative lectures, but this was the best.'

Beyond the pandemic, the urgent question now is: how quickly can the Indian economy rebound? Neelkanth Mishra, co-head of APAC Strategy and India strategist for Credit Suisse, looked ahead[42] as the pandemic waxed and waned:

> 'Now that there is evidence of high levels of seroprevalence in the population, with nearly 80 per cent of the most vulnerable (those above 45 years of age accounted for 90 per cent of Covid deaths) having antibodies, it is time to look at India's economic output in a full year without any activity restrictions.
>
> 'In economic forecasting, trend is a good friend: In "normal" times, collective human behaviour tends to be somewhat predictable. The reason why estimates of economic output from different firms are so remarkably close is not just the innate human urge to conform ("herd behaviour" among forecasters), but also that economies have a certain momentum which persists unless some external forces are applied, not unlike the "objects in motion" that Newton described in his laws. Imagine an upward sloping line (called the "trend line"). The economic output (GDP) of a country tends to fluctuate around it. If trend growth is 6.5 per cent, growth in a year tends to be between 6 and 7 per cent, and most forecasts would be in that band. Without a significant shock, growth rarely moves outside it. Trend lines also change over time, but usually this is not a sudden change.
>
> 'Can there be a problem of demand? Given that the pandemic has left many lower-income households with higher debt and/or fewer assets, their consumption maybe constrained. However, not only is much of their demand non-discretionary, in aggregate, the bottom half of households only consume as

[42]The *Indian Express*, 22 July 2021.

> much as the top 10 per cent. The latter have been left with elevated financial savings, some of which are likely to be spent in the coming months. Improving penetration of personal loans can further support consumption by all types of households.
>
> 'The output post-restrictions is, thus, likely to bounce much higher than currently expected. However, it will still be meaningfully below the pre-pandemic path, and policymakers must look to close the gap. A district or better, block-wise seroprevalence study would give local administrations the confidence to open up schools and transportation, particularly where seroprevalence levels are already above 80 per cent, and focus vaccination efforts where they are not. Thereafter, the recovery may be accelerated by triggering the expenditure of the surplus savings of the rich on labour-intensive services (like travel) or goods (like apparel), say via a shortlived cut in indirect taxes.'

Mishra wrote this at the end of July 2021. By the end of the year, economic output had leapt ahead of pre-pandemic levels. Professor Gagandeep Kang, meanwhile, preferred to place India's battle with Covid-19 within a scientific framework[43]:

> 'We have had SARS-CoV-2 for around 2 years. The original Wuhan virus underwent the D614G mutation and spread rapidly across the world from February 2020. After that we saw no major changes until December 2020, when the Alpha and Beta variants were recognised as increasing rapidly in the UK and South Africa, respectively. Why was there such a gap? Why did significant variants come up in such rapid succession after December 2020, even though the variants' signature mutations had been recognised earlier?

[43]*The Times of India*, 22 July 2021.

> 'One theory, partially borrowed from influenza, is that a certain proportion of the population needs to have been infected for there to be enough immune pressure for the virus to change. Since RNA viruses mutate all the time, mutations begin to matter when there are fewer people to infect. A virus that can overcome the immune response that prevents binding of the spike protein to its receptor or bind to other proteins of the host cell, will be more "fit" and infect more people than a less fit variant. From the point of view of public health, this is a race between the virus and immune systems. If we can protect ourselves with masks, ventilation and limited interactions, until vaccination coverage is above 70 per cent and adds to the protection from prior infection, we can definitely delay or decrease and possibly avoid the next wave.'

Like most analyses, this too can be overtaken by events: future waves could impact newer demographics, including children. Hence Chahal's continuing focus on paediatric facilities in the 11 Jumbo hospitals. The symptoms of 'long Covid' are also a serious problem patients continue to face. Studies have found that those who have recovered after experiencing severe symptoms of Covid-19 often witness a decline in cognitive ability.

The Lancet's EClinical Medicine journal studied 81,000 people to assess the impact[44] of long Covid. Adam Hampshire, who led a team of researchers at London's Imperial College wrote: 'Our analyses provide converging evidence to support the hypothesis that the Covid-19 infection is associated with cognitive deficits that persist into the recovery phase.'

Research teams at Oxford University and the University of Texas have arrived at similar conclusions. Older patients are at particular

[44]*Hindustan Times*, 11 August 2021.

risk of losing cognitive ability after recovering from Covid-19. It is an issue that Indian medical researchers will need to study further even as the vaccination rollout continues.

Scientists have long debated the longevity of infectious viruses. K. Srinath Reddy, an epidemiologist who is president of the Public Health Foundation of India, notes[45]:

> 'Cautionary counselling, that we should not sound militaristic calls for microbial eradication in our response to infectious agents, comes from a scientist who won the Nobel Prize for Medicine and Physiology at a very young age in 1958—Joshua Lederberg. In a seminal essay on the history of infectious diseases, published in *Science* in 2000, he advises us to discard the "waging war" metaphor and recognise the evolutionary imperatives that drive the microbe's behaviour. Lederberg suggests that "a successful parasite (one that will remain infectious for a long time) tends to display just those epitopes (antigenic fragments that stimulate the immune system) as will provoke responses that a) moderate but do not extinguish the primary infection and b) inhibit other infections by competing strains of the same species or other species". Is the Delta variant racing to claim that crown or will yet another variant emerge to achieve a better balance between high infectivity and continued presence among the human population, which it will seek to use for replication but be careful not to extinguish?
>
> 'Why will the virus become less virulent over time? Because its survival advantage depends on having a human host, in whom it can replicate. It cannot afford to wipe out our species, for it will script its own extinction by doing so. Why

[45] *The Indian Express,* 28 August 2021.

> then does the SARS-CoV-2 virus still kill so many across the world? Lederberg's essay provides an explanation. He writes: "Those relatively few infectious agents that cause serious sickness or death are actually maladapted to their host, to which they may have only recently gained access through some genetic, environmental or sociological change." That fits the SARS-CoV-2 virus so well! The virus can still be made to adapt through human strategies.'

Chahal follows the science governing Covid-19 with interest. He processes the information and uses relevant parts in his numerous public speeches. When Chahal addressed the Young President's Organization (YPO), comprising India's emerging business leadership, he detailed the MCGM's strategy to combat the pandemic and speed up the vaccination drive. Chahal later spoke to the Southeast Asian YPO, regarded as the gold standard among rising young business leaders across the region.

He has also addressed top global business and thought leaders based in Singapore. Says Chahal: 'The Ideas and More Group is an elite group of 300 top business leaders and fund managers across the world who control $600 billion worth of trade and assets. I also addressed the British Business Group, the Indo-Swiss Chamber of Commerce and the Public Concern for Governance Trust led by J.F. Reberio.' Chahal and his work were quoted in August 2021 in the *British Medical Journal* which, he points out, is like being embossed in the long-term memory of medicine, possibly for a century.

But as Chahal and his team at the MCGM know, the battle against Covid-19 will finally be won only by fully vaccinating the country's adult population of 940 million and a large section of the 400 million children below the age of 18. That challenge lies ahead.

TEN

VACCINATING THE NATION

India's vaccination programme got off to a slow start on 16 January 2021. It was only on 21 June when the Centre took over the distribution of vaccine doses after a hiatus in April and May that the pace of inoculation picked up. Several obstacles had to be overcome.

Production capacities at the two local vaccine manufacturers Serum Institute of India (SII) and Bharat Biotech (BB)—took time to ramp up. Tardy payments by the Union government slowed the rollout. Authorisation of foreign vaccines like Russia's Sputnik and local ones such as Zydus Cadilla along with greater quantities of Covishield from SII and BB helped raise administered doses to an average of over 8 million per day. Though the Centre's target of innoculating 100 per cent of India's 940 million adults by 31 December 2021 with two doses of the Covid-19 vaccine (1.88 billion doses in all) was not fully met, India's vaccination drive has proved to be an overall success. Chahal is confident that despite latent vaccine hesitancy, Greater Mumbai is well on its way to become the first major Indian metropolis to achieve close to full inoculation of adults.

'Two years ago, when the first wave hit us in March 2020,' says Chahal, 'there were obviously no vaccines available for the novel coronavirus. Vaccines for new viruses take years to develop. It is rare to produce a safe and efficacious one in less than 10 months as Oxford-AstraZeneca and Pfizer, among others, did for Covid-19. It was a great challenge for scientists worldwide to create an effective vaccine to counter Covid-19. Even clinical trials and processes for new vaccines often take as long as 7-8 years before they are approved. Here time was running out for mankind. We needed a vaccine in months, not years, given the scale of deaths and infections caused by Covid-19.'

By the end of 2020, there was a ray of hope that an effective and safe vaccine would become a reality in the near future. Researchers at Oxford University's Jenner Institute led the way with successful clinical trials. The British government's Medicines and Healthcare Products Regulatory Authority (MHRA) approved Oxford-AstraZeneca's vaccine for adults in the United Kingdom in December 2020, allowing Britain a head start in vaccinating its adult population and eligible children under 18.

India produces 60 per cent of the world's vaccines. It supplied Pulse Polio drops to around 60 countries and is the largest single global manufacturer of vaccines. The Serum Institute of India, based in Pune, has long been a world leader in vaccinations. Says Chahal: 'It was very reassuring to us. We had faith in Serum Institute. Mass production soon began at its Pune plant. Trials for Covishield were held in many places all over the world, including at MCGM hospitals. Covishield is identical to the Oxford-AstraZeneca vaccine that is being manufactured and used under licence in several countries.

'At around the same time, another indigneous company from Hyderabad, Bharat Biotech, researched, developed and manufactured Covaxin. Trials for Covaxin were conducted at many places in the country, including all MCGM hospitals in Mumbai. Similarly, companies like Pfizer, Johnson & Johnson, Moderna, Sputnik in Russia and Sinovac in China, developed their own vaccines.'

In India, the National Vaccination campaign, the largest anywhere in the world, bar China, covered 1.38 billion people. The government decided that in the first phase, beginning on 16 January 2021, health workers would get priority and be the first to get inoculated. 'Mumbai has approximately 1,50,000 health workers,' Chahal points out. 'So we started the vaccination drive with them. The arrival of a safe and effective vaccine was a great relief for the entire world. Countries had been suffering from Covid-19 for nearly a year. From 4 February 2021, the union government added frontline workers to the vaccine priority list. Health workers are primarily doctors and paramedical staff. Frontline workers include ambulance drivers, ward boys, support staff in hospitals and MCGM employees. This was phase two of the vaccination rollout.

'We have 3,00,000 frontline workers in Mumbai. The target for phase two was these frontline workers. We made rapid progress. We started administering 40,000 vaccine doses per day. A number of private hospitals were included in this drive. There was, however, initial vaccine hesitancy. We found that even health and frontline workers were hesitant to take a vaccine dose. I had to conduct meetings with private hospitals to urge them to promote the vaccination campaign. On one particular day, of a total of 45,000 vaccines administered, MCGM hospitals accounted for 41,000 doses and private hospitals for only 4,000.'

The union government announced that phase three of the vaccine rollout would commence from 1 March. It was decided that all citizens above the age of 60 and citizens above the age of 45 who had comorbidities would be covered in this phase. Says Chahal: 'In the first wave, we had found that major mortalities were from those above 60 years. Immunity obviously declines with age while comorbidities increase. As the second wave tightened its grip over India, the government extended vaccination to all those above the age of 45, with or without comorbidities. By then we had over 65 vaccination centres in the city. Most of these centres were set up by the MCGM. Finally, on 1 May 2021, it was announced by the union government that all adults above the age of 18 would be covered. This represented a major shift in the vaccination policy of the Centre. Meanwhile, some states advocated that the vaccination rollout would advance faster if it was decentralised, giving states the responsibility for managing the inoculation process.'

A series of policy flip-flops followed. The decentralised policy proved a failure. The number of doses administered per day fell off the cliff. Shortages abounded. Recriminations between the Centre and the states increased. Just when the second wave was at its lethal peak in May 2021, India's vaccination rollout seized up. Dismayed, the prime minister went on national television on 7 June to announce yet another policy shift—this time with greater clarity and decisiveness.

Modi declared in his televised address[46]:

> 'The Centre supervised vaccination from 16 January to the end of April. State governments then said that the Centre should not be allowed to run the vaccination programme. A section of the media ran it as a campaign too. The Union government decided that if this was the thinking, then as an experiment, the states should be allowed to procure vaccines up to 25 per cent from 1 May.
>
> 'States soon became familiar with the challenges of procuring vaccines. Within a fortnight, several states started saying that the earlier system was better. Even those who had most vociferously asked for state procurement fell in line. We thought about it and now it has been decided that there will be vaccine procurement only by the Centre and it will be implemented in the next 2 weeks.
>
> 'The 25 per cent procurement in the hands of the states will be back with the Centre and free vaccines will be available

[46]Translated excerpt, *The Hindu,* 21 June 2021.

for the 18-44 age group too. Crores of Indians have received free vaccines so far. Now those between the age of 18 and 44 will get it for free as well. Those who want to get the vaccine at a private facility, that too has been kept in mind. Private hospitals can only charge ₹150 maximum as service charge over the cost of the vaccine; 25 per cent of the manufacturers' stock will be available for private hospitals. Till now 130 crore Indians have walked together in this battle against Covid. That will continue as we speed up the rate of vaccination. We should remember that our rate of vaccination is faster than many other countries and our tech platform, CoWIN, is also being appreciated.'

A month before Modi's speech, Chahal reveals that he had approached the chief minister. 'On 6 May, I had made a very convincing argument to the CM,' he says. 'I told him that since the time Covid started in Mumbai last March, we have been spending ₹200 crore every month on treatment of patients, running these huge Jumbo hospitals, medicines, housekeeping, catering, electricity bills, pathology labs, salaries to a large number of doctors, etc. So I suggested to the CM that we spend this money on vaccines instead. Covaxin was available for ₹600 per dose, Sputnik for ₹800, Covishield for ₹400. I told the CM that we have a choice: either we spend several hundred crore rupees on the medical ecosystem or we spend that money on procuring vaccines globally and catalysing our vaccination drive. At that time, the Union government had given states a mandate of 50 per cent independent vaccine procurement. Modi had not yet made his 7 June speech.

'On 11 May after discussions with the CM, he gave me permission to go ahead with international bidding. We were the first entity in the country to float a global bid for the procurement of 10 million doses of a vaccine. Any manufacturing company in India or abroad was welcome to participate. We had given 7 days for the global bid which we extented to 25 May. Before 25 May, we got 9 bids. These bids included Pfizer and AstraZeneca. There were 7 bids for Sputnik. In the midst of negotiating with these companies, we had to be very careful. It was something we were dealing with for the first time. These negotiations went on till the last week of May and carried into the first week of June. But all 9 bids were somewhat suspect. We kept on struggling with the bidders who were based in London, Hyderabad and indeed all over the world. The Pfizer bidder was based in the Czech Republic. We told all of them to establish through a legal document, their relationship with the manufacturing company. Unless they gave us documentary evidence of their relationship with the manufacturing company, we could not proceed. Unfortunately no bidder was able to produce a document which would certify that a particular supplier was an authorised distributor or agent of the vaccine manufacturer.

'While this struggle was going on, the prime minister went live on TV on 7 June. He announced that the country would go back to the original centralised protocol but with a small rider. The new protocol would be that 75 per cent of procurement of vaccines would be done by the Union government and it would supply these free of cost to everybody. At the same time, like the 1 May 2021 order, the Union government would keep 25 per cent stock of vaccines for private hospitals. This was a major difference. Prices of various vaccines were announced as well. This protocol would come into force from 21 June. So we cancelled all the international bids. The Centre had made a commitment that we would get vaccines free of cost. The full population above the age of 18 was covered. There was no way we could have a parallel purchase procedure and unnecessarily spend money.'

The MCGM's target is to fully vaccinate 100 per cent of adults in Mumbai by March 2022 even as the drive to inoculate children takes off and gathers pace. Research has shown that even after a single dose of vaccine, mortality rates fall. Serious illness or hospitalisation is rare. This will mitigate the effect of future waves. And yet obviously, neither the city nor the country can afford to let its guard down as it did, with fatal consequences, after the first wave. Concurs Chahal: 'For future waves, we have built new Jumbos. We have built new oxygen plants. I don't rule out a new wave. We are well prepared to handle it.'

The Union government, meanwhile, announced that workplaces and corporate houses which have an ambulance link could do vaccinations outside of designated vaccination medical centres. Mumbai's civic body swung into action. 'We issued orders that all Covid Vaccination Centres (CVCs), especially private hospitals, could literally create a tsunami of vaccinations in Mumbai,' says Chahal. 'We created 400 centres; 120 private hospitals came on board. All these centres gave portable access. We went to the chief justice of the Bombay High Court. The court had called me regarding vaccination of all High Court staff. So we checked and found that there were 2,100 high court staff, from junior staff to the chief justice. We told the HC to give us a list of its employees.

'Now the nearest hospital to the Bombay High Court is Cama Hospital. We decided to park an ambulance in the premises of the high court. We requested the court to give us a large hall. We came with the vaccines and administered the first dose to all the court employees. On one day we administered 1,100 doses and on another day 1,050 doses. We covered the entire high court staff with the first dose of the vaccine. The second dose followed later as per protocol. This workplace vaccination model was again unique to Mumbai. Under this policy you could procure vaccines locally. Reliance Industries procured several lakh vaccines and all these vaccines went to their workplaces: Reliance Industries, Reliance Retail, Reliance Jio, etc. They vaccinated all their employees through portable access. With this idea, 400 vaccination centres could become 4,00,000 centres, depending on the stock of vaccines you have and the ambulance-workplace link.'

Mumbai has several lakh housing societies. On a single day, with an ambulance link, there can theoretically be a large number of vaccination centres. Says Chahal: 'You just needed an ambulance link and a big hall. So we issued a circular that any corporate house, any workplace, any housing society should go to the local or private hospital and sign an MOU with them. The MOU will say that the workplace would provide space and the hospital would provide vaccines and paramedical staff along with an ambulance. Once the MOU is signed they have to inform the MCGM office. They can then go ahead with the vaccination. This is how the nagar sevaks are doing vaccination camps and reaching people who are otherwise hesitant to go to a vaccination centre. Here we are coming to their doorstep with full medical precautions and staff.'

The 2,100 staff in the Bombay High Court received their second dose of vaccines in August. As Chahal says cheerfully: 'Nobody, not the government of India, not the government of Maharashtra, questioned us. We did not violate any of the protocols. We created an ambulance link, assigned a hospital, went to workplaces, and thereby stepped up the vaccination rollout.'

The next challenge was to vaccinate those who were bedridden. Chahal deployed an innovation here as well. 'These people are paralytic or seriously ill,' he says. 'They cannot move out of their beds. How do we vaccinate them? Petitions were filed in the Bombay High Court but this issue could not be resolved. We started a survey of our own and found that there are 4,500 people in Mumbai who are permanently bedridden. We went to the state government and told them to give us this project. It is a huge exercise as we had to go to each of their homes. Suppose in one building only one person is paralysed. We had to go there with an ambulance, along with oxygen equipment.

We had to be in the patient's house for half an hour to monitor him after vaccination. But I said we will do it. From 2 August, we started home-to-home vaccination. Again this was a first in the country. I salute my team for doing this job as it took a lot of effort and time to organise things and move door-to-door. These people are scattered in 4,500 places everywhere, in high-rise buildings and in slums. We filed an affidavit in the Bombay High Court that we are going to do this. Pune and Mumbai carried out this project in Maharashtra. Bedridden patients are not able to go to hospitals, or join vaccination camps, or mass vaccination processes. MCGM teams vaccinated 100 bedridden patients a day and completed the task in record time by the end of September 2021.'

While Mumbai found it easier than other cities to inoculate the adult population under the MCGM's jurisdiction, vaccine hesitancy was evident in small pockets of the city. After the deadly second wave though, vaccine hesitancy declined significantly. Chahal agrees: 'Vaccination hesitancy was present in a big way before the second wave. When I would tell private hospitals that they were vaccinating only 4,000 people per day instead of 45,000 in Mumbai, they would reply that people are just not coming forward for vaccination. But when the second wave hit the country, it eliminated a substantial amount of that hesitancy. People now knew that it was a choice between life and death and that the vaccine could be a saviour. Before the second wave started, the hesitancy was at a level of nearly 50 per cent. Now it has dropped significantly. We have to educate everybody that if you do not ensure 100 per cent vaccination in a city like Mumbai, non-vaccinated people can be a threat to other citizens of the city and, when they travel, to citizens in the rest of the country.

'I approached film personalities like Salman Khan to campaign in favour of vaccination. He was good enough to film a video for us.

It went viral on so many platforms. We are very grateful that he has done the video absolutely free for the MCGM. In the video he said his entire family is vaccinated. So there is no reason why anyone should not take a vaccine dose. He also said if citizens want to save their lives and the lives of their families, they must get vaccinated. This video had an impact. We also worked with more than a dozen NGOs in Dharavi to promote the vaccination drive. Together, we have motivated people and removed a large part of their vaccine hesitancy.'

Challenges, though, remained. One was safe local transportation. To get suburban trains moving again with vaccinated passengers, Chahal suggested a photo identity pass for those with two-dose certification. The CM embraced this solution as local train travel moved the city towards a semblance of normalcy. The advantage of a certified vaccine photo ID pass also encouraged train commuters to become eligible for it by getting themselves vaccinated with both doses.

'This is a weapon I used to remove vaccine hesitancy,' says Chahal, 'and to get commuters back on suburban trains as well. People know that the only way to get the railway photo ID pass is to get vaccinated. Many have got fully vaccinated just to be able to use suburban trains which are vital to their livelihoods. Further, we passed orders that shopping malls, shops, restaurants, gymnasiums, spas, etc. could open up in Mumbai provided their employees were fully vaccinated. Only fully vaccinated citizens could be their customers. This was strictly enforced over the next few months. It proved to be a game changer to crush vaccine hesitancy in Mumbai.'

What of the future? Chahal turns thoughtful as he says: 'We are building 16 new hospitals. I instructed my people to issue floating tenders for all 16 hospitals minus the equipment. New buildings will come up for all the hospitals. The infrastructure of the Jumbos, including advanced medical equipment, will be given to the 16 new hospitals for their new buildings. The MMRDA ground at BKC where our large Jumbo hospital is located, was meant for exhibitions. It is also reserved partly for the proposed bullet train. It will be given back to the MMRDA depending on how things unfold in future waves of Covid-19. But I personally believe that by the first half of 2022, the world would have largely overcome the pandemic which will become endemic like many other viruses we live with.

'We have several sister cities around the world: Los Angeles and New York in the US, Stutgart in Germany, St. Petersburg in Russia, Busan in South Korea and Yokohoma in Japan. We remain in touch on issues of common interest, including, quite obviously, dealing with the Covid-19 pandemic and its aftermath.'

With vaccinating all children under 18 the key focus in 2022, delivering a safe and effective vaccine for this critical demographic has gained momentum. Zydus Cadilla's India-developed ZyCov-D vaccine for children between the ages of 12 and 18 was the first to receive emergency use approval from regulators. It was also the first DNA-based vaccine for Covid-19. As one report[47] described it: 'The vaccine uses a section of genetic material from the virus that gives instructions as either DNA or RNA to make the specific protein that the immune system recognises and responds to. Plug-and-play tech, on which the plasmid DNA platform is based, can be easily adapted to deal with mutations. The shot is given using a needle-free applicator as opposed to a syringe, which will help reduce side-effects.

While future Covid-19 waves may be less lethal following the vaccination rollout, the government is taking no chances. Despite falling demand, it has built a buffer stock of over fifteen critical medicines, including anti-viral Remdesivir, antibiotic Tocilizumab and black fungus drug Amphotericin B. States have access to this buffer stock as well as to new oxygen capacities and special paediatric facilities.

[47]The *Times of India*, 21 August 2021.

'By the first quarter of 2022,' says Chahal, 'Mumbai had vaccinated 99 per cent of eligible citizens with a single dose and 90 per cent with a double dose. At over 99 per cent single dose, Mumbai again led major Indian cities. All eligible citizens would have been fully vaccinated by the end of March 2022.

'Mumbai's vaccination drive has another unique feature. In 5 months, from May 2021 to September 2021, Mumbai administered 98.6 lakh doses of vaccine out of which 46.1 lakh doses were administered by private Covid Vaccination Centres (CVCs). Moreover, 10 lakh vaccines, procured by private hospitals at a cost of nearly ₹65 crore were administered in Mumbai's slums free of cost with CSR funding organised by me and my team from corporate houses.

'Minister Aaditya Thackeray played the role of captain to the team in this initiative. He was the brain behind the CSR funding initiative and used his goodwill to help Team MCGM with more than one million doses of vaccines. But for him, the MCGM's mission of fully vaccinating all its eligible citizens would have taken much longer. He convinced Reliance Industries, Singhania Group, Citibank, HDFC Bank, Godrej and many other corporate houses to liberally donate CSR funds to ensure free vaccination in the slums of Mumbai. He inaugurated various vaccination camps in the slums by personally remaining present despite having suffered from Covid in the recent past. I admire his courage and proactive approach. He has proved to be a problem-solver for the MCGM and never shies away from challenges which confront him. I admire him for the extraordinary qualities which he possesses. He is an ever-smiling personality and a bundle of positive energy. I congratulate him for being a true Covid warrior.

'This quickly catapulted Mumbai to the top position among major cities in India with the administration, to nearly all eligible citizens, of two doses of the vaccine, an important step to fight a third wave in Mumbai triggered by Omicron. We are indebted to corporate and private hospitals of Mumbai. The financial capital of India has shown the way to the nation once again.'

Bill Gates strikes an optimistic note: 'The Melinda and Bill Gates Foundation is very proud that back in the spring of 2020 we gave $300 million to Serum (Institute of India). Serum has executed very well on ramping up the volume, making really record numbers of vaccines. Now that the world understands its vulnerability to a pandemic, there will be a huge amount of research and invention of new tools. The diagnostics—we could scale that up much faster. The therapeutics—we could do a lot better. We should have a goal that we have so much factory capacity that even within 200 days, we could make enough vaccines for the entire world.

'Will this work be ready for the next pandemic, and will it have benefits beyond the pandemic preparedness? The answer is, absolutely yes. For the next pandemic, we will make sure we have gigantic mRNA factories in India and the rest of the developing world to achieve our goal of being able to make vaccines for everyone.'

Chahal mirrors Gates' optimism and ambition. He says simply: 'We will be ready.'

J. LUIS CORREA
46TH DISTRICT, CALIFORNIA

WASHINGTON OFFICE
2301 RAYBURN HOUSE OFFICE BUILDING
WASHINGTON, D.C. 20515
(202) 225-2965

SANTA ANA DISTRICT OFFICE
2323 N. BROADWAY, SUITE 319
SANTA ANA, CA 92706
(714) 559-6190

Congress of the United States
House of Representatives
Washington, DC 20515

HOUSE COMMITTEE ON HOMELAND SECURITY
SUBCOMMITTEE ON OVERSIGHT, MANAGEMENT, AND ACCOUNTABILITY
CHAIR
SUBCOMMITTEE ON BORDER SECURITY, FACILITATION, AND OPERATIONS
HOUSE COMMITTEE ON THE JUDICIARY
SUBCOMMITTEE ON IMMIGRATION AND CITIZENSHIP
SUBCOMMITTEE ON CRIME, TERRORISM, AND HOMELAND SECURITY
HOUSE COMMITTEE ON AGRICULTURE
SUBCOMMITTEE ON LIVESTOCK AND FOREIGN AGRICULTURE
SUBCOMMITTEE ON CONSERVATION AND FORESTRY
SUBCOMMITTEE ON BIOTECHNOLOGY, HORTICULTURE, AND RESEARCH

PROBLEM SOLVERS CAUCUS
BLUE DOG COALITION
NEW DEMOCRAT COALITION
CONGRESSIONAL HISPANIC CAUCUS

July 01, 2021

Dear Commissioner Iqbal Singh Chahal:

On behalf of my constituent, I became aware of Commissioner Iqbal Singh Chahal's great work to help fight the COVID-19 cases in India. It is always great to hear of leaders stepping up to the plate to help others, especially during these unprecedented times.

It is with great appreciation and admiration that I, along with my constituents, recognize your commendable initiatives in the management of the coronavirus pandemic under your jurisdiction in Mumbai.

We commend the various steps you have taken to combat COVID-19 including; Ward level war rooms, integrated hospital bed management through electronic dashboards, individual screenings by doctors at the very beginning of virus infection to prioritize treatment and hospitalization for the needy, and above all your dexterous oxygen supply management. All of the aforementioned accomplishments are hallmarks of your superb managerial skills and astute organizational efficiency rooted in your dynamism and foresight.

Your exceptional strategy brought the COVID-19 positivity ratio from thirty percent in the beginning of April, down to just four percent today - which speaks volumes for your accomplishments.

We extend our heartiest congratulations and best wishes to you for your continued success in serving your constituents during the pandemic in Mumbai. You are a true role model for your junior colleagues in the civil service.

Respectfully,

Lou Correa
Member of Congress

CORREA.HOUSE.GOV

LIST OF AWARDS/ APPRECIATION/RECOGNITION

Sr. No.	Award Name	Year of Award	Field	Type of Award	Awarding Authority
1.	Letter of Appreciation	2021	Spectacular performance in fight against Covid	Others	Grouping comprising of retired Cabinet Secretaries of India and retired Chief Secretaries of State
2.	Newsmakers Achievers Award	2020	Best IAS Officer - Covid Pandemic Management	National	Afternoon Media Group
3.	Letter of Appreciation and Admiration	2021	Exceptional Covid Management and Control Strategy	International	Sitting Member of Congress, USA, Washington
4.	Qimpro Medal	2021	Establishment of benchmark in Covid Management	National	Qimpro Foundation, India
5.	The Sakaal Sanmaan Award	2021	Outstanding Performance in Covid Pandemic	State	Sakaal Media, Pune

6.	India Business Leader Award (IBLA)	2021	Covid Pandemic Management and Control	National	CNBC-TV 18 Network
7.	SKOCH Covid Champion	2021	Exemplary Performance in Covid Management	National	SKOCH Group, India
8.	Citizen of Mumbai Award	2021	Covid Pandemic Management and Control	Others	92 years old Rotary Club of Mumbai
9.	Covid Crusader Award	2020	Covid Pandemic Management and Control	International	Indo American Chamber of Commerce
10.	Mumbai Ratna Award	2021	For saving thousands of lives in Covid Pandemic	State	Regd. HRD, Government of India
11.	India's Distinguished IAS Officer	2021	Covid Pandemic Management and Control	National	SpeakIn, Asia's largest on demand expert network (SpeakIn)
12.	Maharashtrian of the year	2021	Stellar Performance in Covid Pandemic control	State	Lokmat Trust, Nagpur
13.	Iconic Achiever's Award	2021	Stellar Performance in Covid Pandemic control	National	WBR Group, New Delhi

14.	Certificate of Recognition	2021	Exemplary leadership and excellence in crisis management of Covid-19 in Mumbai	International	The Consul General of Spain in Mumbai, India

INDEX